CHEMISTRY AND FUNCTIONS OF COLICINS

ACADEMIC PRESS RAPID MANUSCRIPT REPRODUCTION

Proceedings of a Conference on The Structure and Functions of Colicins, at the 72nd Annual Meeting of the American Society for Microbiology, Held in Philadelphia, Pennsylvania, May 1972

CHEMISTRY AND FUNCTIONS OF COLICINS

edited by
LOWELL P. HAGER
Department of Biochemistry
School of Chemical Sciences
University of Illinois at Urbana-Champaign
Urbana, Illinois

Academic Press, Inc.
NEW YORK AND LONDON

A Subsidiary of Harcourt Brace Jovanovich, Publishers

ACADEMIC PRESS, INC.
111 Fifth Avenue, New York, New York 10003

United Kingdom Edition published by
ACADEMIC PRESS, INC. (LONDON) LTD.
24/28 Oval Road, London NW1

Library of Congress Cataloging in Publication Data
Main entry under title:

Chemistry and functions of colicins.

"Proceedings of a conference on the structure and functions of colicins, at the 72nd annual meeting of the American Society for Microbiology, held in Philadelphia, Pennsylvania, May 1972."

1. Colicins–Congresses. I. Hager, Lowell P., ed. II. American Society for Microbiology. [DNLM. 1. [DNLM: 1. Colicins–Congresses. 2. Colicins–Pharmacodynamics–Congresses. QV350 A512c 1972]
QP801.C7C47 615'.329'95 72-88348
ISBN 0–12–313550–8

PRINTED IN THE UNITED STATES OF AMERICA

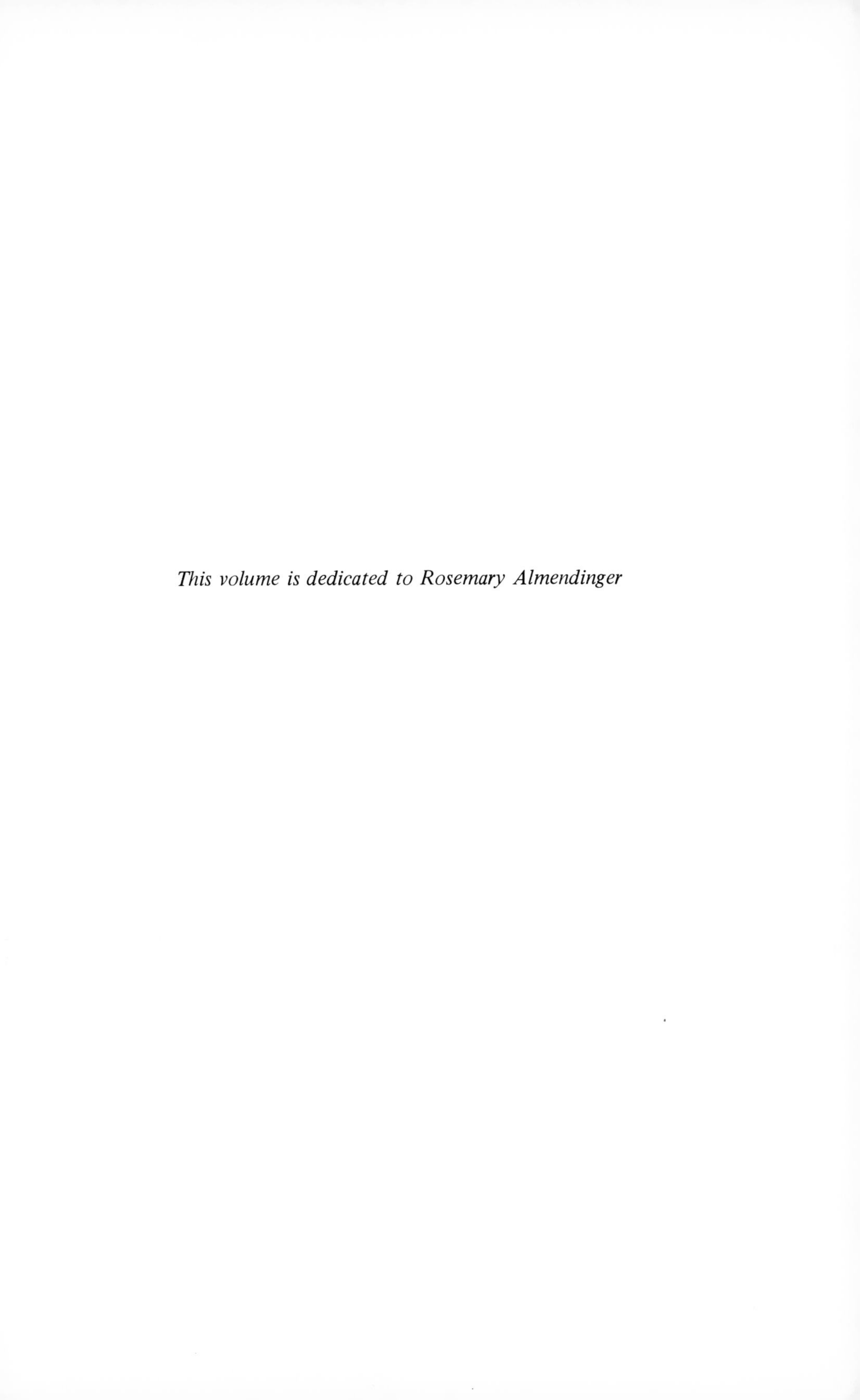

This volume is dedicated to Rosemary Almendinger

CONTENTS

CONTRIBUTORS

Rosemary Almendinger
Enzyme Institute, University of Wisconsin Medical School, Madison, Wisconsin 53706

C. Michael Bowman
University of Wisconsin Medical School, Madison, Wisconsin 53706

Lowell P. Hager
Department of Biochemistry, University of Illinois, Urbana, Illinois 61801

Donald R. Helinski
Department of Biology, University of California at San Diego, La Jolla, California 92037

Jordan Konisky
Department of Microbiology, University of Illinois, Urbana, Illinois 61801

S. E. Luria
Department of Biology, Massachusetts Institute of Technology, Cambridge, Massachusetts 02139

Joan Lusk
Department of Chemistry, Brown University, Providence, Rhode Island 02912

Masayasu Nomura
Enzyme Institute, University of Wisconsin Medical School, Madison, Wisconsin 53706

C. A. Plate
Department of Biology, Massachusetts Institute of Technology, Cambridge, Massachusetts 02139

Sohair F. Sabet
Department of Biology, Massachusetts Institute of Technology, Cambridge, Massachusetts 02139

Carl A. Schnaitman
Department of Microbiology, School of Medicine, The University of Virginia, Charlottesville, Virginia 22901

J. Sidikaro
Enzyme Institute, University of Wisconsin Medical School, Madison, Wisconsin 53706

PREFACE

The colicin field continues to offer a fertile field for studies concerning the chemistry and molecular biology of cell surfaces, control of macromolecular synthesis and energy coupling. The recent dramatic discovery of an *in vitro* enzymatic activity for colicin E_3, the new findings concerning the role of RNA in the replication of col factor E_1, the reconstitution of E_2 induced DNA degradation in spheroplasts, and the isolation of colicin receptors open yet a new series of chapters in the colicin story. The contributions recorded in this book represent the latest and in most instances previously unpublished work from several laboratories which have concentrated on quite different aspects of colicinology. This material was first presented in a symposium entitled "The Structure and Function of Colicins," at the 72nd annual meeting of the American Society for Microbiology in Philadelphia, May 1972. The contributors to this symposium kindly provided typescripts of their presentations and these were skillfully prepared for printing by Miss Connie Ogden.

I wish to take this opportunity to thank the contributors for their efforts to bring this volume to a successful conclusion. I especially commend them for their patience and perseverance during a long winter of indecision.

Lowell Hager

CHEMISTRY AND FUNCTIONS OF COLICINS

COLICINS

S. E. Luria, Joan Lusk, C. A. Plate

Abstract

A brief statement on the history of colicin research, introducing recent advances on the action of various colicins on sensitive cells, is followed by a summary of the authors' studies with colicins E_1 and K. Two early stages in the action of these colicins are defined. The second stage is characterized by damage to membrane-associated cellular functions, resembling the effects of chemical uncouplers but distinct from them in significant respects. It is suggested that the inhibition of protein synthesis may be at least partly secondary to the inability of colicin E_1-treated bacteria to retain amino acids.

The fortunes of certain research areas seem to fluctuate like the stock market. When Gratia (1) discovered colicins in 1925 there was a minor flurry of excitement, then silence, or rather background-level noise for almost 40 years. The findings that some colicins killed sensitive cells by a single-hit kinetics and arrested macromolecular syntheses likewise stirred little interest. Colicin research came of age when Nomura and his co-workers (2) as well as other groups discovered that different colicins had distinct biochemical effects and that some of these effects could be overcome by the action of trypsin on colicin-treated cells.

If that was a coming of age for colicin research, the present Symposium may celebrate a wedding. In the last year some adolescent fantasies of colicin research have been set aside and a fruitful union of genetic, biochemical and enzymatic approaches has taken place. Yet, even in this more settled state, colicin research remains a very exciting field for people interested in membranes and transport phenomena.

Some properties of colicin molecules and of the corresponding colicinogenic factors are presented in Table I and the key findings on colicin action are listed in Table II. The isolation of colicin-resistant mutants indicated the existence of specific colicin receptors. That trypsin can partially restore viability to a colicin-treated culture suggests that the colicin, following adsorption to its receptor, remains susceptible to proteolytic attack for some

Table 1

Colicins and Colicinogenic Factors

Colicin	Mol. wt.	f/f_o	Isoel. point	Col factor DNA
E_1	56,000	2.02	9.05	4.2×10^6
E_2	60,000	(1.41)	7.63, 7.41	5×10^6
E_3	60,000	(1.41)	6.64	5×10^6
K	70,000	-	5.7	-
I	79,000	1.8	-	-

Table 2

General Characteristics of Colicin Action

1. Viability loss follows first order kinetics (one-hit).
2. Viability can be partially restored by trypsin.
3. Certain bacterial mutants (resistant) lose ability to adsorb specific groups of colicins.
4. Different colicins cause different biochemical effects.

period of time. The one-hit kinetics indicates that one (successful) colicin molecule can kill a cell. On the basis of these and other findings Nomura (2) proposed the model outlined in Table III. The key

Table 3

Nomura's Model

1. Attachment of colicin to receptor site.
2. Reversible change at attachment site.
3. Transmission of change to the "target".
4. Effects on biochemical and killing target.

feature of the model, postulated to reconcile trypsin reversibility with biochemical damage, was the idea of a mechanism that conveys the stimulus generated by colicin at its receptor site to a biochemical target by an action transmitted through (and possibly also along) the cytoplasmic membrane.

Several recent developments have both amplified and modified the picture embodied in this model. The other papers in this Symposium deal with most of these exciting developments. Sabet and Schnaitman (3) have isolated what appears to be receptor proteins for some colicins and have shown that the bulk of these substances are in the external cell-wall layer of the *Escherichia coli* envelope. That the effective receptors may be a minority located in the membrane has not yet been excluded.

The most remarkable advances have been at the level of colicin action. Dr. Bowman's paper in this Symposium will describe how Boon (4) and soon thereafter the Nomura group (5) discovered that colicin E_3, which causes a delayed arrest in protein synthesis, produces a direct damage to the 16S ribosomal RNA when mixed with ribosomes *in vitro*. Whether the colicin does this by an enzyme activity of its own or by activating some ribosomal enzyme is still unsettled.

Progress has been made also in the study of colicin E_2, which *in vivo* leads to progressively increasing DNA damage. Almendinger and Hager (6) have proposed an intriguing hypothesis of colicin E_2 action on intracellular DNA through displacement of the endoplasmic space. Whether colicin E_2 has an endonucleolytic activity of its own has not been excluded. It would be surprising if two colicins like E_2 and E_3, similar in molecular size and shape, serological reactivity and receptor specificity, were to act in perversely different ways, one as an enzyme, the other as the agent for displacing an enzyme within the bacterial cell. But, at any rate, it is clear that some features of Nomura's original model have to be modified.

Our own recent work, which will be summarized in the remainder of this paper, concerns primarily colicins K and E_1, both of which inhibit macromolecular syntheses (2) as well as a variety of active transport processes coupled to electron transfer (7; see Table 4). The first question to which we address ourselves is the reversibility of the action of these

Table 4

Effects of Colicins K and E_1

Inhibition of biosyntheses (protein, nucleic acid, glycogen...)
Inhibition of cellular motility
Inhibition of accumulation of amino acids, β-galactosides...
No inhibition of accumulation of α-glucosides

colicins. Nomura and Nakamura (8) found that treatment with trypsin caused a return of viability and resumption of protein synthesis in *E. coli* B cells that had been treated with colicin K. In our experiments with *E. coli* K-12 we have used trypsin in an attempt to define successive stages in the action of colicins K and E_1 and the kinetics of the transitions between these stages. More specifically, we have asked whether one can, on the one hand, determine the proportion of cells that, already complexed with col icin, have not yet manifested physiological damage and, on the other hand, the proportion of cells that are still rendered viable by a given trypsin treatment. Then we have asked what the relationship is between the two. If the two proportions are the same we would conclude that the trypsin treatment rescues only those cells without manifest physiological damage. Figure 1 illustrates this possibility (hypothesis A) together with the alternative (hypothesis B) that the trypsin treatment can restore both viability and function.

The experiments consisted of adding trypsin to cell-colicin complexes at various times and measuring viable counts on the one hand and transport or protein synthesis on the other hand. Typical results are shown in Figures 2 and 3. In all cases the addition of trypsin after a delay of one or two minutes prevented further effect of colicin on the retention of a substrate or on the incorporation of an amino acid into protein. In all cases the residual levels of function corresponded precisely to the fraction of cells whose viability had been preserved by trypsin (Figure 4). There was no sign of recovery of

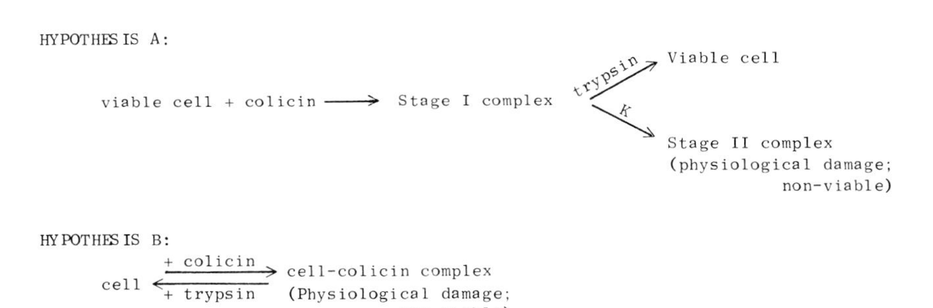

Figure 1 - Trypsin Reversal of Colicin Action

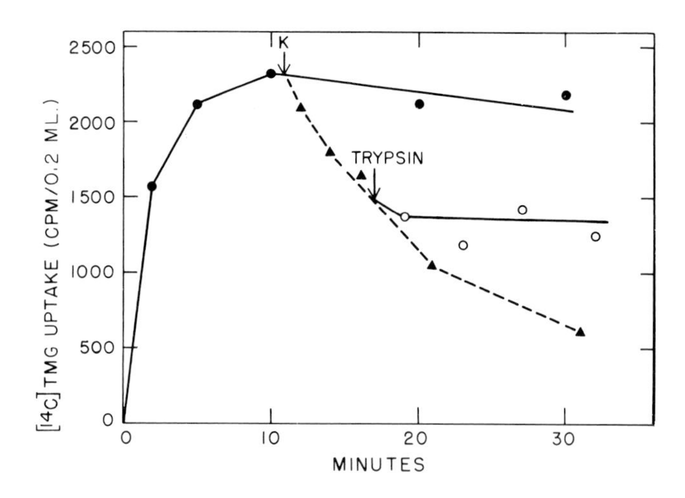

Figure 2 - Effect of trypsin on colicin K-induced efflux of thiomethyl-β-D-galactoside (TMG). Washed cells of E. coli strain LA319 lac^- ($i^-z^-y^+$) grown in a lactate medium and placed at 27° received [1-^{14}C]-TMG (10^{-4} M· 2.5 μCi per mole). Aliquots of 0.2 ml were collected on filters, washed, and counted. Colicin K (about 2 killing units) and trypsin (500 μg/ml final concentration) were added to samples of the culture at the indicated times. Bacterial survival measured immediately before addition of trypsin was 0.21; survival after 15 minutes of trypsin treatment was 0.57.

function even when observation was continued up to one hour (Figure 3).

We interpret these findings as evidence in favor of hypothesis A of Figure 1: trypsin treatment as practiced in our experiments can render viable only those cells in which no damage has yet been caused by colicin K. We define as Stage I the condition in which attached colicin has not yet manifested its physiological action and Stage II as that period during and following colicin action. Note that these experiments were successful because we used low multiplicities of colicin.

What is the Stage I → Stage II transition?

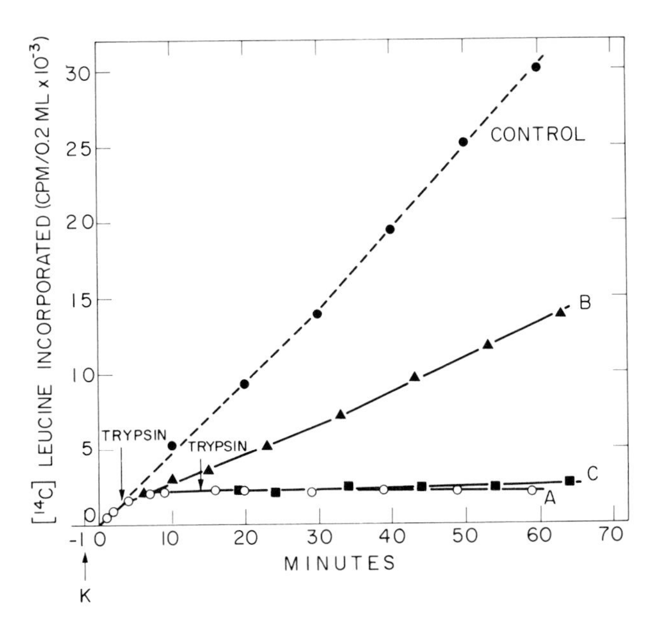

Figure 3 - Effect of colicin K and trypsin on protein synthesis at 27°. Cells of E. coli LA319 received [U-^{14}C]-leucine (10^{-4} M· 10 μCi per mole). Culture A received colicin K one minute before leucine, and samples from it received trypsin (500 μg/ml) 4 minutes (B) or 15 minutes (C) after addition of colicin. Aliquots of 0.2 ml were transferred to trichloroacetic acid and the precipitates were collected, washed, and counted. Bacterial survival was 0.63 in sample B and 0.10 in sample C 15 minutes after addition of trypsin.

Figures 5 and 6 illustrate experiments with colicins K and E_1 showing that rescuability by trypsin decays with time at an exponential rate. This rate is temperature dependent (Q_{10} about 3) and, more important, is directly proportional to the "killing multiplicity" of colicin, that is, to the maximum number of effective hits that a given amount of colicin would produce in the absence of trypsin. We interpret this to mean that each "potentially killing" colicin molecule

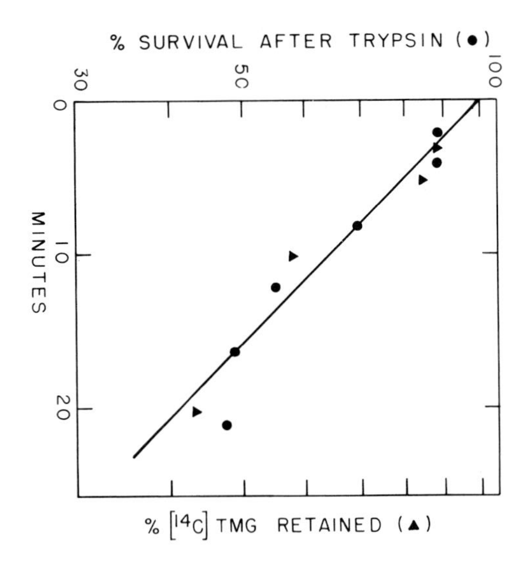

Figure 4 - Ability of colicin K-treated cells to form colonies and retain TMG when trypsin is added at various times after colicin. LA319 cells were incubated with [1-^{14}C]-TMG at 27° until a steady state level of accumulation was reached (10 min); then colicin K was added. At the indicated times portions of this culture were either treated with trypsin and plated for survival, or were used to measure TMG retention as described in the legend to Figure 2. Survival without trypsin treatment, measured 5.5 min. after colicin K addition, was 28 per cent.

(presumably, a molecule adsorbed to a specially located receptor) has a constant probability per unit time to pass from Stage I to Stage II, independently of the action of other colicin particles. Wendt (9) has also concluded, on the basis of studies on the exit of potassium ions from colicin K-damaged cells, that attached colicin K molecules do not act in a cooperative fashion.

Once colicin reaches State II, cellular damage follows. We have not yet succeeded in dissociating Stage II, defined by the occurrence of functional

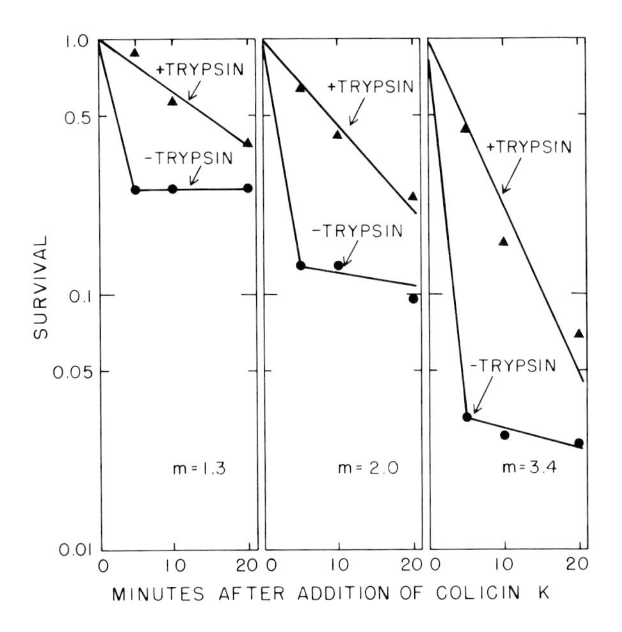

Figure 5 - Effect of trypsin on colicin K-induced loss of viability. LA319 cultures (5×10^8 per ml) were treated for 5 min. at 27° with different concentrations of colicin K and were then diluted 10-fold to decrease further adsorption. Colicin K concentration is expressed as multiplicity (m), determined from the equation $S/S_o = e^{-m}$ where S/S_o is the survival ratio. At various times after colicin addition, aliquots were either diluted and plated or were incubated with trypsin (500 μg per ml; 15 min; 27°) prior to plating. Survival was determined after overnight incubation of the plates at 37°.

damage, from a possible Stage II-A, in which reversibility by trypsin ends but functional damage has not yet taken place. The experiments of Nomura and Nakamura (8) in which protein synthesis could be restored by trypsin to K-treated cells indicate a significantly different situation. Experiments in progress should serve to resolve this discrepancy.

The next question is whether the various effects

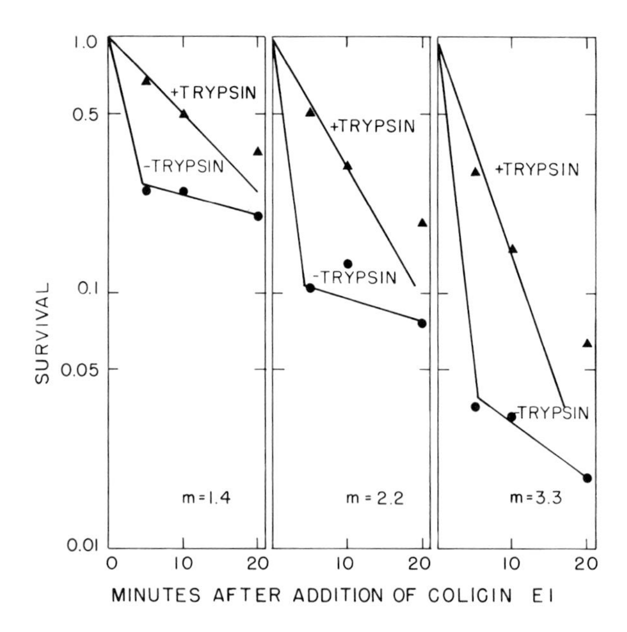

Figure 6 - Effect of trypsin on colicin E_1-induced loss of viability. Experimental details were the same as described in the legend to Figure 5, except that colicin E_1 was used.

of colicins K and E_1 are independent or are sequential manifestations of colicin action. Recent experiments have led us to the conclusion that the arrest of protein synthesis by colicin E_1 is subsequent to, and possibly is in part the consequence of, the colicin-initiated inhibition of amino acid transport. When the colicin is added first and then the incorporation of exogenous labeled amino acids into proteins is measured, this incorporation stops promptly, within 2 to 5 minutes after addition of colicin. But in experiments like that shown in Figure 7, in which the amino acid pool was preloaded for a few minutes with a labeled amino acid before adding colicin E_1, incorporation into protein continued for a few minutes longer and ceased only when the amino acid pool was greatly reduced. Many factors other than the dimin-

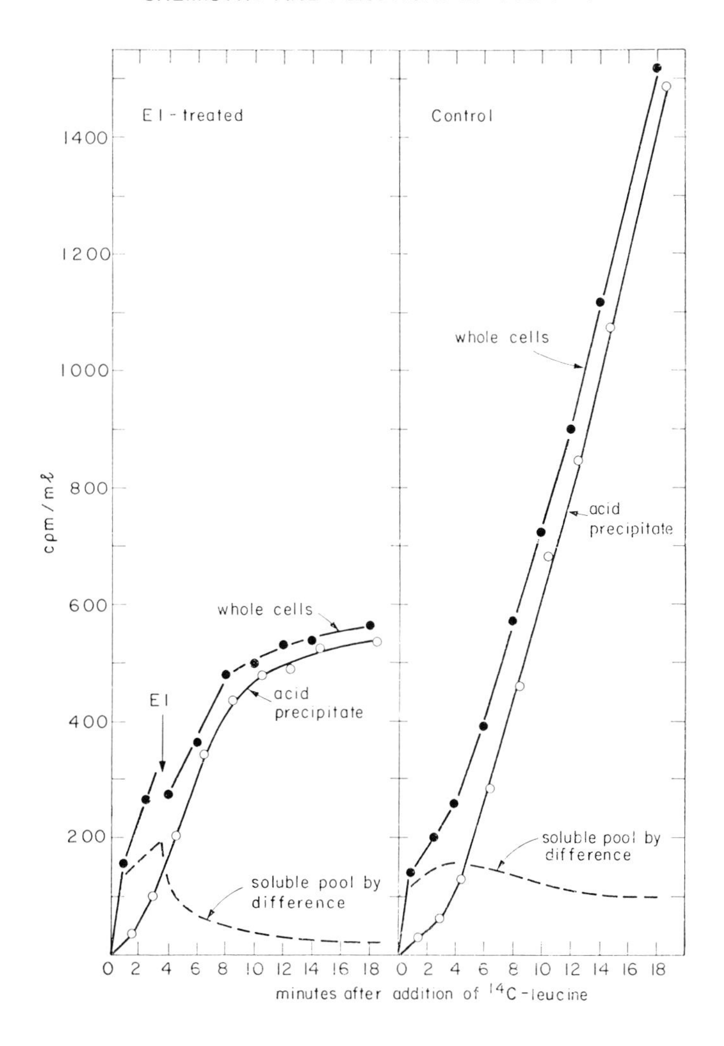

Figure 7 - Effect of colicin E_1 on accumulation and incorporation of leucine. Cells of E. coli C600 leu^- grown in supplemented glucose minimal medium were washed and resuspended in cold medium base. At zero time a 1:24 dilution was made in medium containing [U-^{14}C]-leucine (4.3 μg/ml; 0.2 mCi/mg). Colicin E_1 was added to one sample. Uptake of leucine was measured by filtering 0.1 ml aliquots and washing at room temperature. Incorporation into protein plus tRNA was measured on aliquots treated with trichloroacetic

(Figure 7, cont'd) acid. The free leucine pool was taken to be the difference between total uptake and incorporation. Bacterial survival was 1.6 per cent at 1.5 minutes and 0.08 per cent at 20 minutes after addition of colicin E_1.

diminished pools of amino acids, including lack of m-RNA and reduced ATP levels, certainly contribute to the inhibition of protein synthesis. This experiment, however, clearly suggests that transport, a process intimately associated with the membrane, is inhibited by colicin E_1 before protein synthesis is affected.

The effects of colicins E_1 and K on various transport systems are summarized in Table 5. Besides

Table 5

Effects of colicins K and E_1 on membrane exchanges

EFFECT	K	E_1	CCCP FCCP
Inhibition of TMG accumulation	+	+	+
" αMG "	-	-	-
" amino acid "	+	+	+
Leakage of glycolytic intermediates	+	+	-
Promotion of H^+ entry		-	+
Inhibition of Mg^{++} exchange	+	+	+
Promotion of Mg^{++} efflux	+	(+)	-
" " Co^{++} entry	+	(+)	-
" " K^+ efflux	+	+	-

the fact that not all transport systems are inhibited (hence the permeability barrier is not grossly damaged) the main finding is that the effects of K and E_1 can be distinguished from those caused by the chemical "uncouplers". Uncouplers facilitate entry of protons into cells, presumably by acting on the lipid bilayer (10). Colicin E_1 does not cause proton entry (11). Instead, both K and E_1 cause efflux of K^+ and Mg^{++} ions (9,12). In addition these colicins cause an influx of Co^{++} ions into an *E. coli* mutant that cannot transport Co^{++} and is relatively impermeable to this ion (12). Such ion movements are not observed upon treating *E. coli* with chemical uncouplers. The conclusion, not fully documented here, is that these effects on ion efflux and influx are exerted, not just through inhibition of active transport systems, but in part through what appears to be a specific damage to the membrane. In colicin K-treated cells damage becomes evident after a lag whose duration depends on temperature and on multiplicity of colicin. In contrast, the inhibition of accumulation of substrates like galactosides or amino acids is observed quite rapidly after addition of colicin. We take, therefore, as a working hypothesis that colicin K and probably also E_1 exert on the cytoplasmic membrane of sensitive cells a series of effects representing either progressive damage to certain membrane components or a damaging action extending successively to different membrane components. The fact that one particle of colicin can successfully carry out the damaging actions without cooperativity suggests a localized damage that spreads from one site of primary action. The most promptly manifested effects on transport may be exerted through an inhibition of the system described by Kaback (13) that couples D-lactate oxidation to active transport.

Many important questions remain to be answered. Is the primary action of colicin on the cytoplasmic membrane enzymatic or conformational? If enzymatic, is the damage to membrane components caused directly by the colicin or indirectly through bacterial enzymes? Which membrane components are primarily affected -- proteins, phospholipids, or others? Students of colicins are probably justified in believing that the investigation of the action of these proteins will provide novel and exciting insights into the functional organization of the bacterial membrane.

References

1. Gratia, A. (1925) C. R. Soc. Biol. 93, 1040.
2. Nomura, M. (1963) Cold Spring Harbor Symp. Quant. Biol. 23, 315.
3. Sabet, S. R., and Schnaitman, C. A. (1971) J. Bacteriol. 108, 422.
4. Boon, T. (1971) Proc. Natl. Acad. Sci., U. S. 68, 2421
5. Bowman, C. M., Sidikaro, J., and Nomura, M. (1971) Nature New Biol. 234, 133
6. Almendinger, R., and Hager, L. P. (1972) Nature New Biol. 235, 199.
7. Fields, K. L., and Luria, S. E. (1969) J. Bacteriol. 97, 57.
8. Nomura, M., and Nakamura, M (1962) Biochem. Biophys. Res. Commun. 7, 306.
9. Wendt, L. (1970) J. Bacteriol. 104, 1236.
10. Hopfer, U., Lehninger, A. L., and Thompson, T. E. (1968) Proc. Natl. Acad. Sci., U. S. 59, 484.
11. Feingold, D. S. (1970) J. Membr. Biol. 3, 372.
12. Lusk, J. E., and Nelson, D. L. (1972) J. Bacteriol. (in press).
13. Kaback, H. R. (1970) Ann. Rev. Biochem. 39, 561.

CHEMISTRY OF COLICINOGENIC FACTORS

Donald R. Helinski

Studies on the chemical properties of the genetic determinants of colicin production, termed colicinogenic (Col) factors, have provided considerable information on the variety of structures that extrachromosomal elements assume in the host bacterial cell. The various DNA forms and DNA-protein complexes of *Col* factors that have been described have given also some insight to the chemical basis of *Col* factor replication, the conjugal transfer of these elements and the expression of colicin production. *Col* factors, as in the case of other stable extrachromosomal elements (plasmids) in bacteria, can be classified into two major genetic types on the basis of the presence or absence in the element of genetic determinants of sexuality. Of the colicinogenic factors considered in this presentation, *Col*E_1, *Col*E_2, and *Col*E_3 do not carry the determinants for sexuality in bacteria. The conjugal transfer of these factors requires the presence of a sex factor plasmid present in the same cell. *Col*V and *Col*Ib are plasmid elements that are designated sex factors since these plasmids promote their own transfer or the transfer of the host chromosome to a female cell. These two *Col* factors can be further categorized into F-type and I-type sex factors on the basis of the determination of an F-type pilus by the *Col*V plasmid and an I-like pilus by the *Col*Ib element. In this communication a consideration of the chemical properties of these various types of colicinogenic factors will be carried out within the framework of plasmids in general. Particular attention will be focused on the possible implications of the chemical properties of *Col* factor DNA and complexes of *Col* factor DNA and protein with respect to our understanding of plasmid replication and the conjugal transfer of plasmids from donor to recipient cells.

General Properties of Col Factors

Recent advances in our understanding of the physical chemical properties of circular DNA (1) have enabled the development of several techniques that greatly facilitate the extraction of Col factor DNA from the host cell and the purification of this plasmid DNA (2, 3). Table I summarizes the properties of Col factors that have been purified in our laboratory by dye-cesium chloride equilibrium centrifugation and sucrose density gradient sedimentation procedures.

TABLE I

Structural Properties of Col factors Isolated from E. coli*

Col factor	Sex-factor type	Colicin determined	Molecular weight	Covalently-closed circular DNA	No. copies per chromosome	References
$ColE_1$	None	E_1	4.2×10^6	+	10-15	3,4
$ColE_2$	None	E_2	5.0×10^6	+	10-15	3
$ColE_3$	None	E_3	5.0×10^6	+	10-15	3
ColV**	F	V	94×10^6	+	1-2	5
FColVColBtrycys	F	V and B	107×10^6	+	1-2	6
ColIb	I	Ib	62×10^6	+	1-2	7

* Parent strains of the various colicinogenic factors are as follows (in parenthesis): $ColE_1$ (K-30); $ColE_2$ (Shigella sp. P9); $ColE_3$ (CA38); ColV (K94); FColVColBtrycys (YS57); and ColIb (Salmonella typhimurium L2 cys D36); unless otherwise noted, the parent strains are E. coli.

** Studies with ColV in our laboratory were carried out by Ron Leavitt.

The use of the dye-cesium chloride equilibrium centrifugation technique takes advantage of the covalently-closed circular form of double stranded Col factor DNA, the natural state of the majority of Col factor molecules in the host cell. As shown in Table I, the Col factors lacking sex factor properties ($ColE_1$, $ColE_2$ and $ColE_3$) are of a relatively low molecular weight and are present to the extent of many copies (10-15) per copy of chromosome. Both the F-type and I-type *Col* factors sex factors are of a relatively high molecular weight and are present to the extent of 1 to 2 copies per copy of chromosome. Although in the case of each *Col* factor the majority of the molecules are in the covalently-closed, circular, duplex DNA (supercoiled) form, the presence of a substantial percentage of the supercoiled *Col* factor DNA molecules in the form of a relaxation complex of supercoiled DNA and protein precludes the use of the dye-cesium chloride buoyant density technique for the complete recovery of *Col* factor DNA as supercoiled DNA since this procedure induces a relaxation (conversion to the open-circular or nicked DNA form) of the complex supercoiled DNA (8). In addition the quantitative recovery of the *Col* factor-sex factor plasmids in the form of supercoiled DNA is difficult due to the greater shear and endonuclease sensitivity of these relatively high molecular weight elements during extraction (breakage of a single phosphodiester bond results in the loss of superhelicity in a covalently-closed molecule (9)). Figure 1 is an electron micrograph of the covalently-closed (supercoiled) and the open circular DNA forms of the colicinogenic factor *FColVColBtrycys*.

Multiple Circular DNA forms of *ColE*$_1$

The presence of the majority of the *Col* factor molecules described in Table I as a monomer circular DNA form in *E. coli* is not the case for the *ColE*$_1$ element after this plasmid has been transferred to a foreign host, *Proteus mirabilis*. A substantial proportion of *ColE*$_1$ DNA molecules extracted from logarithmically growing *P. mirabilis* are in the dimer and trimer molecular weight supercoiled forms (10). The addition of chloramphenicol to a growing culture of *P. mirabilis* (*ColE*$_1$), or amino acid starvation of these cells, results in an accumulation of higher multiple (tetramers, pentamers, etc.) supercoiled

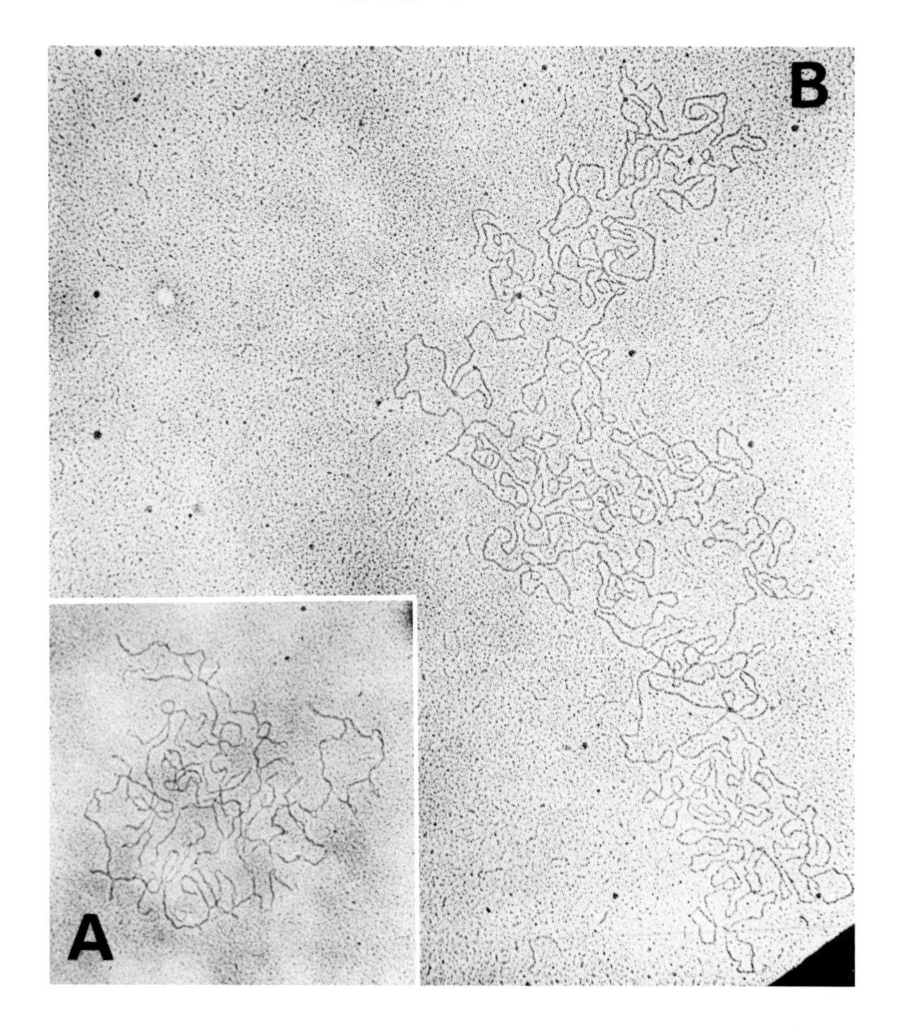

Figure 1 - Electron micrographs of the DNA of the plasmid FColVColBtrycys purified by preparative cesium chloride equilibrium centrifugation. (a) Supercoiled DNA form. (b) Open circular DNA form. The scale line represents 1.0μ. (From Hickson *et. al.* (6)).

forms (10). Figure 2 is an electron micrograph of higher multiple supercoiled DNA forms isolated from *P. mirabilis* ($ColE_1$) cells grown in the presence of

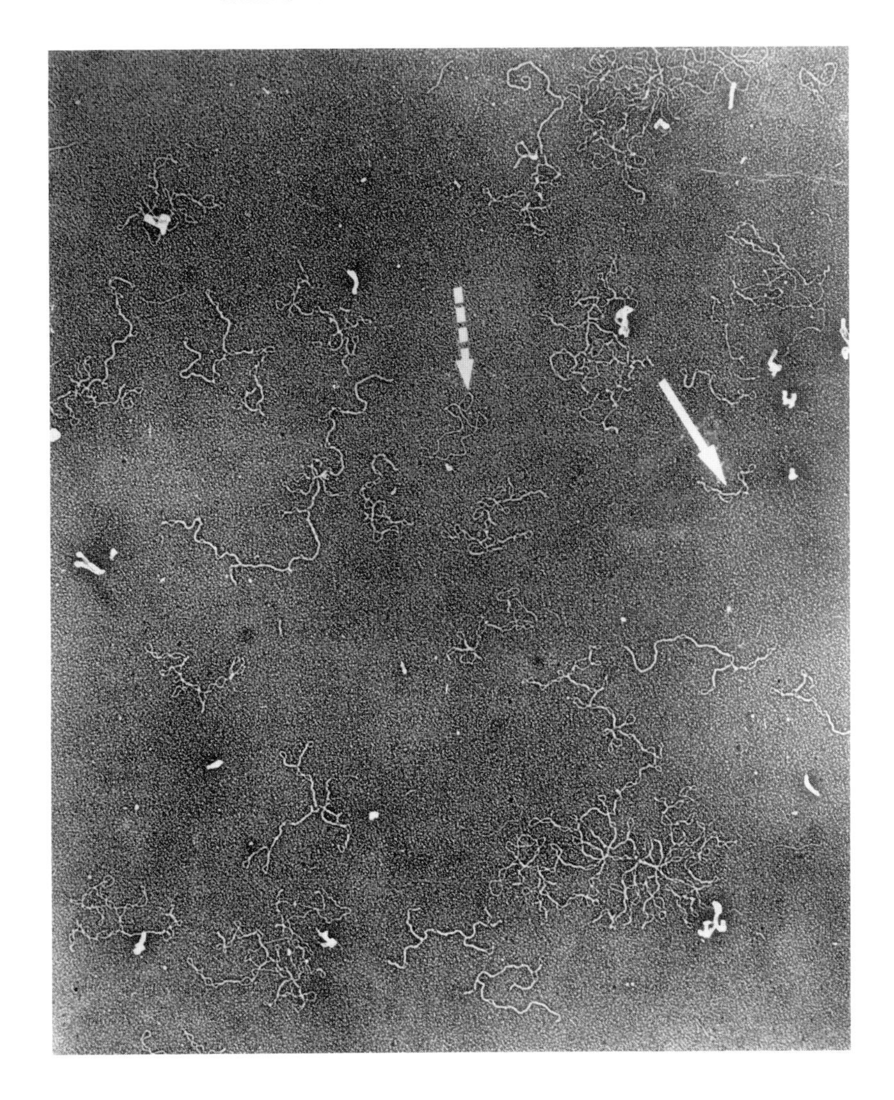

Figure 2 - Electron micrograph of the DNA of the plasmid ColE$_1$ synthesized in P. mirabilis cells grown in the presence of chloramphenicol. DNA was purified (10) and prepared for electron microscopy (6) as described previously. The intact arrow indicates the supercoiled monomer form of ColE$_1$. The broken arrow indicates the open circular monomer form of ColE$_1$. Other structures include supercoiled multiple circu-

(Figure 2, cont'd) lar DNA forms of ColE$_1$. (W. Goebel and D.R. Helinski, unpublished data).

chloramphenicol. Table II summarizes the properties of ColE$_1$ DNA isolated from E. coli (ColE$_1$) and P. mirabilis (ColE$_1$) cells. On the basis of results of radioisotope labeling of ColE$_1$ DNA during the formation of the higher multiple supercoiled DNA forms, it was proposed that the majority of the multiple circular DNA forms were generated by errors in circular DNA replication in the foreign host rather than by a random recombination process involving a pool of monomer circular DNA molecules (10). A circular DNA replication mechanism was proposed that could be responsible for the replication of ColE$_1$ DNA and the generation of multiple circular DNA forms (Figure 3) (10). A similar mechanism of circular DNA replication also has been proposed by others (see 12) and the designation "rolling-circle" for this mechanism was made by Gilbert and Dressler (13). To date there is no direct evidence in support of a "rolling-circle" mechanism of ColE$_1$ replication. While "circle with tail" DNA forms of ColE$_1$ have been observed in mini-cells of E. coli, these forms are found to a

TABLE II

Properties of ColE$_1$ Plasmid*

	E. coli (ColE$_1$)	P. mirabilis (ColE$_1$)
% of molecules supercoiled	>95%	>95%
Molecular weight	4.2×10^6	4.2×10^6 8.5×10^6 12.7×10^6
Effect of inhibition of protein synthesis	Continued synthesis of monomer copies	Synthesis of monomer, dimer, trimer and higher multiple forms

* References for these observations are (3) (4) (10) and (11).

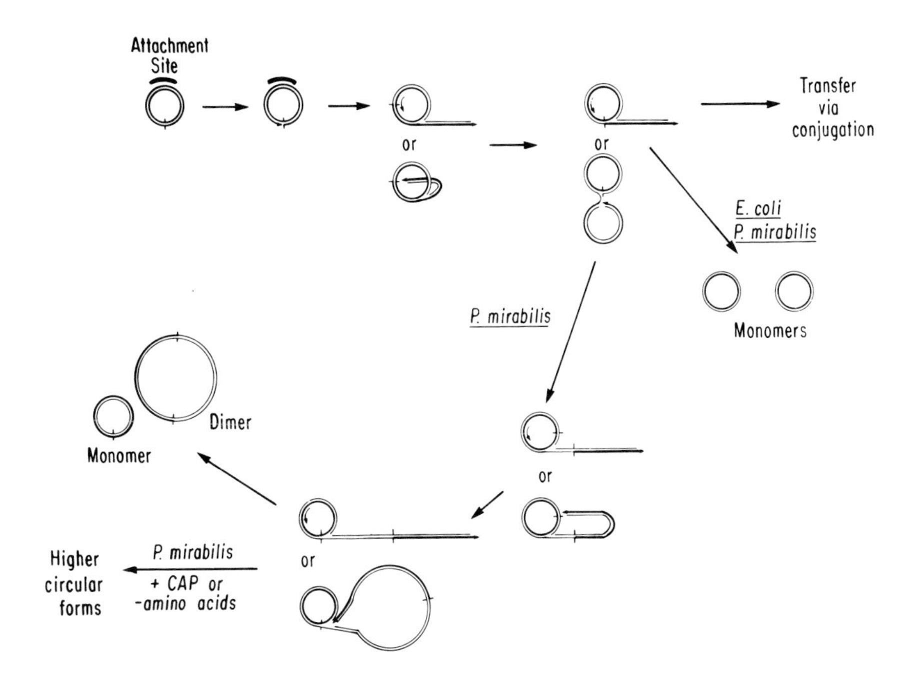

Figure 3 - Model for the formation of higher multiple circular DNA forms. Duplication of the $\underline{ColE}_1$ DNA is considered to involve initially a break in one of the phosphodiester bonds of one of the two strands of the covalently-closed double-stranded circle. During the process of duplication one of the strands remains in the covalently closed cyclic form and serves as a template for the potential synthesis of an unlimited number of covalently-linked complete sequences of the other strand. The failure to carry out a second endonucleolytic cleavage, necessary for the release of the duplicated strand prior to cyclization, after the duplication of one length of circular DNA is considered to occur with increased frequency in P. mirabilis under conditions of inhibition of protein synthesis. The heavy lines represent parental DNA strands, and the light lines represent newly synthesized DNA strands. (From W. Goebel and D.R. Helinski (10)).

considerably less extent than double-forked open circles and covalently-closed, forked circles amongst a population of forked $\underline{ColE_1}$ structures (14).

Col Factor Relaxation Complexes

A number of models have been proposed for the duplication of a circular DNA molecule. While these models differ widely with respect to proposed cyclic intermediates in the duplication process, there is general agreement on the basis of strong theoretical considerations in favor of at least one break in one of the polynucleotide strands during the replication of a covalently-closed circular DNA molecule. It is not clear whether this hypothetical nicking of the supercoiled structure is effected by a single nicking event at a unique site in the molecule, or multiple, non-specific, nicking and sealing events occur during the replication process. Similar considerations can be made for the conjugal transfer of plasmid DNA, where it is clear that at least one nick must occur in the covalently-closed, circular DNA prior to the transfer of a unique strand of this DNA to a recipient cell. A clue to the nature of the nicking event in the replication or conjugal transfer of plasmids may lie in the properties of unusual complexes, termed relaxation complexes, of supercoiled plasmid DNA and protein that have been purified in our laboratory after lysing plasmid-containing E.coli cells with non-ionic detergents (7, 8, 15, 16, 17, 18).

A relaxation complex of Col factor DNA and protein is readily detected by sucrose density gradient analysis of the supercoiled Col factor DNA before and after treatment with an ionic detergent as sodium dodecyl sulfate (SDS) or sodium dodecyl sarcosinate (Sarkosyl), a protease as pronase, or short exposure to alkali (pH 12.5). As shown in Figure 4 after treatment of a mixture of non-complexed supercoiled $\underline{ColE_1}$ DNA and differentially labeled complexed supercoiled $\underline{ColE_1}$ DNA with Sarkosyl or pronase, the major-

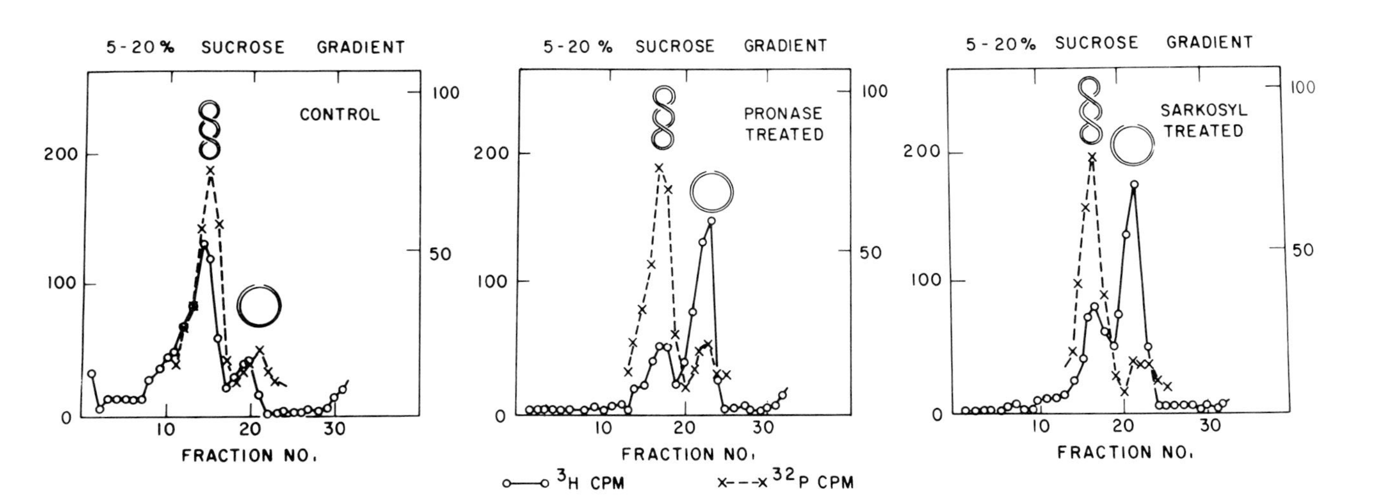

Figure 4 - Sucrose gradient analysis of ColE$_1$ relaxation complex. A mixture of [^{3}H]-thymine-labeled complexed ColE$_1$ DNA and [^{32}P]-labeled non-complexed ColE$_1$ DNA was centrifuged in a 5-20% neutral sucrose density gradient after no treatment (left panel), treatment with 1.25 mg/ml pronase (middle panel), and treatment with 0.25% Sarkosyl (right panel). The position of the supercoiled and open circular DNA forms of ColE$_1$ DNA in the gradients are indicated. The top of the gradient is on the right in each case. (From Clewell and Helinski (8)).

ity of complexed DNA molecules sediment as a slower sedimenting form. The non-complexed supercoiled $\underline{\text{Col}}E_1$ DNA molecules are unaffected by this treatment. In the case of the relaxation complex of supercoiled $\underline{\text{Col}}E_2$ DNA and protein prior heat treatment (60°C, 20 min) renders the relaxation complex essentially insensitive to subsequent treatment with SDS or pronase (17). The heat treatment has been shown to effectively remove the protein from the $\underline{\text{Col}}E_2$ DNA (17). Electron microscopy (Figure 5) and alkaline sucrose density gradient analyses (16, 17, 18) have established in the case of every plasmid complex that has been examined that the product of the SDS or pronase

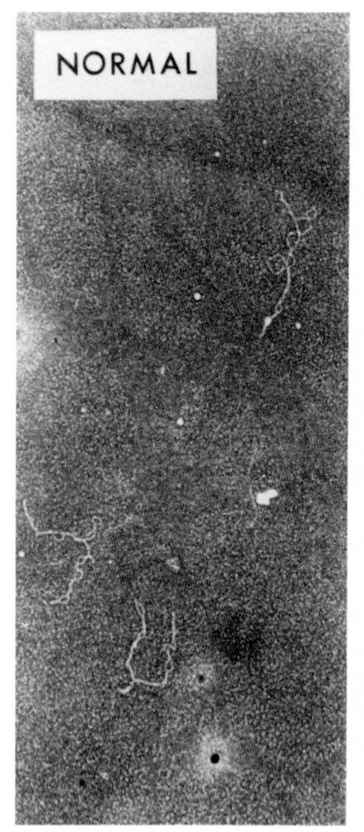

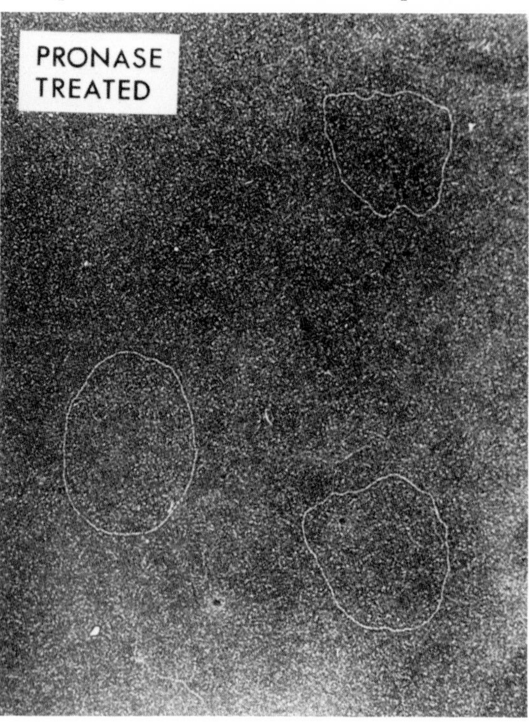

Figure 5 - Electron micrographs of purified complexed $\underline{\text{Col}}E_1$ DNA prior to (left panel) and after treatment with pronase (1.6 mg/ml) (right panel). (From Clewell and Helinski (8)).

induced relaxation event is an open circular DNA molecule possessing a single nick. Utilizing the strand separation technique of cesium chloride equilibrium centrifugation of DNA in the presence of poly-(U,G) (19), the strand specificity of the nicking event in the case of the relaxation complexes of $ColE_1$, $ColE_2$ and the sex-factor F_1, was established (Table III). In the case of each of these three complexes the nicked strand is the heavy strand of DNA

TABLE III

Relaxation Complexes of Supercoiled DNA and Protein

Plasmid	% of molecules complexed	Strand specificity of relaxation event	References
$ColE_1$	15-90*	heavy strand (poly UG)	8, 16, 17
$ColE_2$	20-90*	heavy strand (poly UG)	15, 17
$ColE_3$	70-80	not know	15
ColV	~50	not know	R. Leavitt, unpublished data
ColIb	~80	not know	7
F_1	~50	heavy strand (poly UG)	18

* Extent of $ColE_1$ plasmid molecules in the form of relaxation complex varies with host strain, growth medium and incubation temperature ((11) and L. Katz, D.T. Kingsbury and D.R. Helinski (manuscript submitted for publication)).

as defined by cesium chloride centrifugation in the presence of poly (U,G). It is of additional interest that the nicked strand in the case of the sex factor F_1 is identical to the strand found by Vapnek and Rupp (20) to be transferred to a recipient cell during conjugal transfer of the F_1 plasmid.

The loss of protein and resistance to SDS or pronase as a result of heat treatment *in vitro* of the $ColE_2$ complex argues in favor of the relaxation complex consisting of covalently-closed, circular DNA associated with an inactive, strand-specific, endonuclease that can be activated *in vitro* by agents that induce relaxation (16, 17). On the basis of these observations it is less likely that the supercoiled DNA in the relaxation complex possessed a pre-existing nick with the associated protein functioning as a "binder" of the two termini of the nicked region (16). The heat inactivation of relaxation complex has also been observed in the case of the $\underline{F}_1$ relaxation complex (18). On the other hand the $\underline{Col}F_1$ relaxation complex is not inactivated by heat treatment; rather the supercoiled DNA in this complex is converted to the open circular DNA form by heat treatment (8).

If the relaxation complexes play a role in the early steps of replication and/or conjugal transfer of plasmid DNA, the properties of these complexes would indicate that the initiation of plasmid DNA replication or conjugal transfer involves, at least as part of the process, the activation of a latent endonuclease that catalyzes a nick in a specific strand and possibly at a unique site. In the case of conjugation the broken strand is transferred to the recipient cell. In the case of replication DNA polymerization would ensue, or, if already primed, permitted to continue following the nicking event. To date, however, there is no direct evidence for a role of relaxation complexes in plasmid DNA replication or transfer and the physiological role of these complexes remains to be determined.

Temperature Sensitive Plasmid DNA Replication Mutants

An essential role for DNA polymerase I of *E.coli* in the replication of the $\underline{Col}E_1$ plasmid is clearly indicated from studies in our laboratory with a *polA1* mutant of *E.coli* (21) and an analysis of mutants of *E.coli* that were isolated on the basis of their temperature sensitivity for $\underline{Col}E_1$ replication (Kingsbury and Helinski, manuscript submitted for publication). The *polA1* mutant studies also showed some dependency for the DNA polymerase I enzyme for $\underline{Col}E_2$ maintenance. The maintenance of *Col*V and *Col*Ib was not effected in the DNA polymerase I mutant cells indicating a lack of dependency for this enzyme for the replication of these Col factors.

In addition to the temperature sensitive $ColE_1$ replication mutants that exhibited a temperature sensitive DNA polymerase I, other $ColE_1$ replication mutants have been isolated that possess normal DNA polymerase I activity and are either specific for $ColE_1$ replication or affect the maintenance of other plasmid elements. As shown in Table IV these mutants can be grouped into various categories on the basis of the chromosome or plasmid location of the mutation and the plasmid specificity of the mutation. All of these mutants appear to be normal with respect to chromosomal DNA replication. It is clear from the properties of these mutants that mutations on either the host chromosome or on the $ColE_1$ replication. The plasmid-linked mutations are specific for the replication of the $ColE_1$ factor. The host mutants can be classified into three groups on the basis of the plasmid specificity of temperature sensitive mutants. Mutants of group I are unable to maintain at 43°C any of the six plasmid elements described in Table IV. Group II mutants specifically affect the replication

TABLE IV

Classification of Temperature-Sensitive $ColE_1$ Replication Mutants*

Plasmid**	Sex-factor type	Mutant Class				
		Chromosome located				Plasmid located
		I	II	IIIa	IIIb	
$ColE_1$	None	ts***	ts	ts	ts	ts
Flac, ColV, R1	F	ts	ts	wt	wt	wt
ColIb, R64	I	ts	wt	wt	wt	wt

* Data of Kingsbury and Helinski (manuscript submitted for publication).

** E. coli parent strain of Flac is C6000. R1 (Km, Cm, Sm, Su, Am) and R64 (Tc, Sm) were derived from E. coli strain J5-3. Origin of other plasmids is given in Table I.

*** ts and wt refer to temperature-sensitive and wild-type, respectively.

of the ColE$_1$ and F-type plasmids, but not the I-type plasmids ColIb and R64. Finally, the group III mutants that are specific for ColE$_1$ can be subdivided into group IIIa and IIIb. The group IIIa mutants exhibit a temperature sensitive DNA polymerase I while the group IIIb mutants show normal activity for this enzyme. The temperature sensitivity of DNA polymerase I activity in extracts of two of the group IIIa mutants (TS214 and TS216) is shown in Figure 6. Certain of the mutants in group IIIb plus select mutants

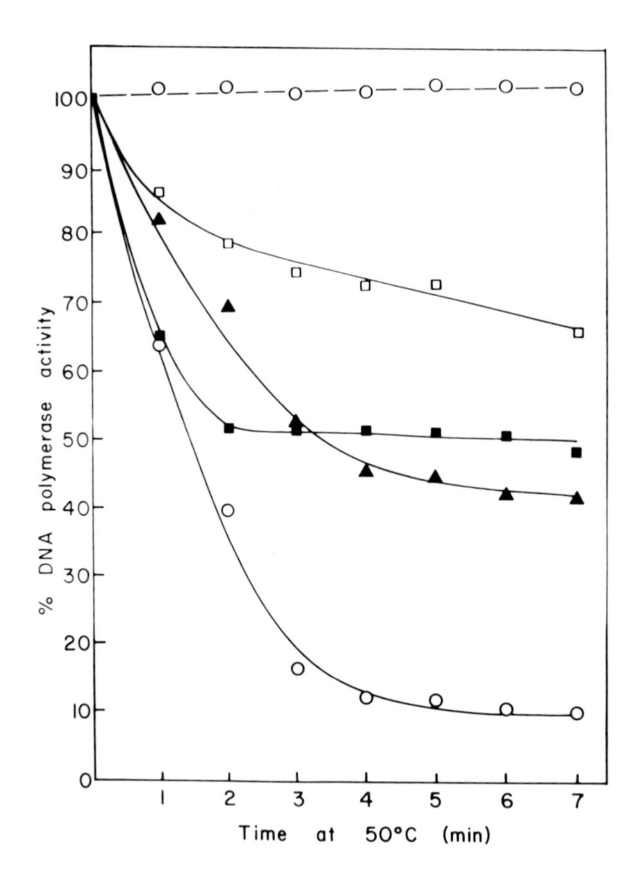

Figure 6 - Thermal sensitivity of DNA polymerase I in ColE$_1$ DNA replication mutants. Brij lysates (8) of control (E. coli DK100), TS214 and TS216 cells were

(Figure 6, cont'd) assayed for DNA polymerase I activity after incubation of the extracts for various periods of time at 50°C. The control and mutant strains are derivatives of the E. coli strain JC411 (ColE$_1$). TS214 and TS216 are temperature sensitive for the replication of the ColE$_1$ plasmid and are classified as group IIIa mutants. (o---o) control; (o——o) TS214; (■——■) 1:1 mixture of TS214 and control extracts; (▲——▲) TS216; (□——□) 1:1 mixture of TS216 and control extracts. (D.T. Kingsbury and D.R. Helinski, manuscript submitted for publication.

of groups I and II show a temperature sensitivity of growth to concentration of deoxycholate that do not affect the growth of the wild-type strain (D.T. Kingsbury, D.G. Sieckmann and D.R. Helinski, manuscript submitted for publication). This suggests a temperature sensitive membrane defect in at least some of these mutants.

In addition to the striking effect of the temperature sensitive mutations on the replication of ColE$_1$, these mutations also result in the temperature sensitive inability of a donor cell to transfer the ColE$_1$ plasmid during bacterial mating (D.T. Kingsbury and D.R. Helinski, manuscript submitted for publication). Similarly, the ColE$_1$ plasmid cannot be transferred or established in a recipient cell carrying the temperature sensitive replication mutation upon mating with a wild-type donor of this plasmid at 43°C. In the few cases examined the plasmid specificity of the mutants for maintenance of the various plasmids was reflected in the plasmid specificity of the mutations towards the transfer of the different plasmid elements.

RNase Sensitive Supercoiled ColE$_1$ DNA

While the precise role of DNA polymerase I in the replication of the ColE$_1$ plasmid is unknown, some insight to the early polymerization events in the replication of this plasmid may be given by recent

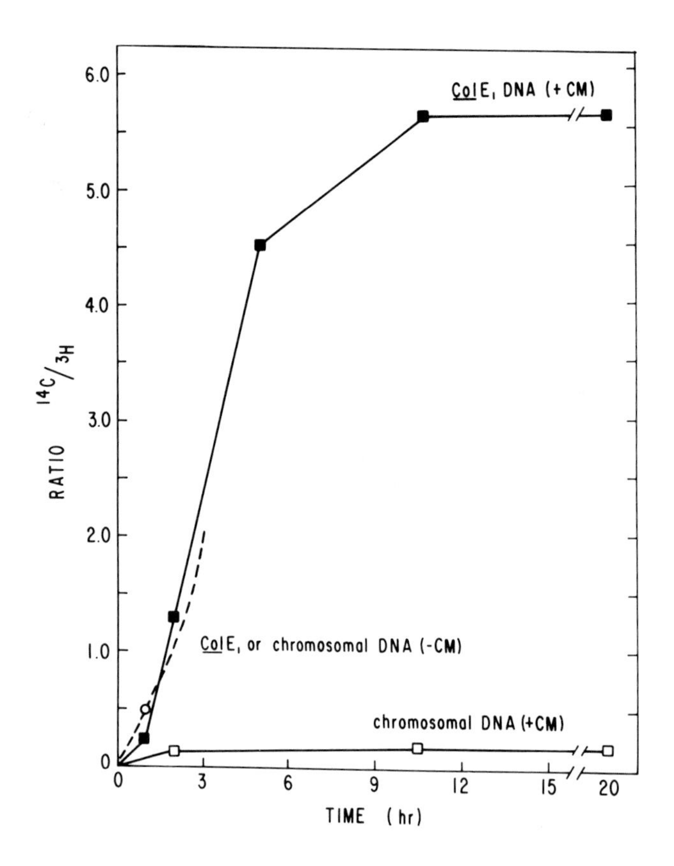

Figure 7 - $\underline{ColE_1}$ DNA synthesis in E. coli cells after the addition of chloramphenicol. JC411 ($\underline{ColE_1}$) cells were labeled with [^{3}H] thymine prior to the addition of CM and with [^{14}C] thymine after the addition of CM (150μg/ml). The single point for the relative DNA synthesis of both plasmid and chromosomal DNA in the absence of CM was determined after 1 generation after [^{14}C] thymine addition. The broken line was drawn assuming an exponential rate of synthesis. (D.G. Blair and D.R. Helinski, unpublished data).

observations on the properties of the $\underline{ColE_1}$ factor DNA synthesized in cells grown in the presence of chloramphenicol. The direct dependence of DNA replication on RNA synthesis has been indicated in several systems with the finding in these cases that DNA synthesis is sensitive to inhibition of RNA synthesis by such RNA polymerase inhibitors as rifampicin and streptolydigin (22, 23, 24, 25). In the case of the conversion of M13 single-stranded phage DNA to the double-stranded RFII form, it has been demonstrated that, at least *in vitro*, RNA plays a role as a primer and is covalently joined to the newly synthesized DNA strand (26). As indicated in Table II $ColE_1$ DNA synthesis continues in *E. coli* cells when protein synthesis is inhibited by the addition of chloramphenicol (CM). Under these conditions chromosomal DNA synthesis ceases within 1-2 hours after the addition of CM, while, as shown in Figure 7, $ColE_1$ DNA synthesis continues for 10 to 15 hours resulting in the accumulation of 1000 to 3000 copies of supercoiled $ColE_1$ DNA per cell (11, 22). The covalently-closed $ColE_1$ DNA synthesized under these conditions essentially consists of protein-free molecules. Furthermore, Clewell *et al.* (22) made the striking observation that plasmid DNA synthesis in the presence of CM is sensitive to rifampicin suggesting a direct role for RNA in the $ColE_1$ DNA replication process. The remaining portion of this presentation will concern itself with the possible relationship of these observations to a unique property of supercoiled $ColE_1$ DNA synthesized in *E. coli* cells in the presence of chloramphenicol.

Electron microscopy, sucrose density gradient and dyecesium chloride buoyant density centrifugation analyses established that $ColE_1$ supercoiled DNA synthesized in the presence of CM (CM-$ColE_1$) is not grossly modified in size, configuration or base composition when compared with $ColE_1$ supercoiled DNA generated in the absence of CM (non-CM $ColE_1$) (27). On the other hand, a substantial portion of $ColE_1$ supercoiled DNA molecules replicated in the presence of CM exhibit a striking sensitivity to alkaline pH conditions. As shown in Figure 8 CM-$ColE_1$ DNA loses its covalently-closed structure upon incubation at pH 13 in phosphate buffer, while non-CM-$ColE_1$ DNA is

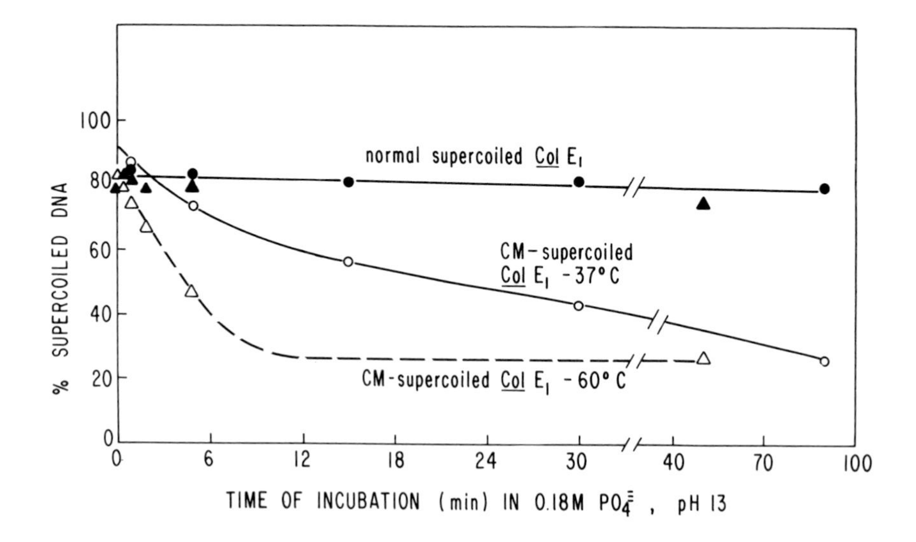

Figure 8 - Alkaline lability of covalently-closed CM-$ColE_1$ DNA. Samples of supercoiled non-CM-$ColE_1$ and CM-$ColE_1$ DNA were incubated at pH 13 in 0.18M PO_4 at the temperatures and for the times indicated, then neutralized and analyzed on 5-20% sucrose density gradients. Supercoiled DNA is expressed as a percentage of total $ColE_1$ DNA recovered from the gradients. (From Blair *et. al*. (27)).

only slightly affected by the alkaline conditions during the time period of the experiment. If the CM-$ColE_1$ DNA is denatured by incubation at pH 13 and 4°C and immediately neutralized there is no significant loss of its covalently-closed structure.

The observations of Clewell *et. al*. (22) with respect to the rifampicin sensitivity of CM-$ColE_1$ DNA synthesis and the role of RNA as a primer in DNA synthesis in the M13 *in vitro* DNA synthesis system (26) raised the possibility that the alkaline sensitivity of CM-$ColE_1$ supercoiled DNA was due to the presence of RNA in these covalently-closed molecules. The sucrose density gradient results, depicted in Figure 9, show that a 10 minute treatment with RNase A of a mixture of differentially labeled CM- and non-CM $ColE_1$

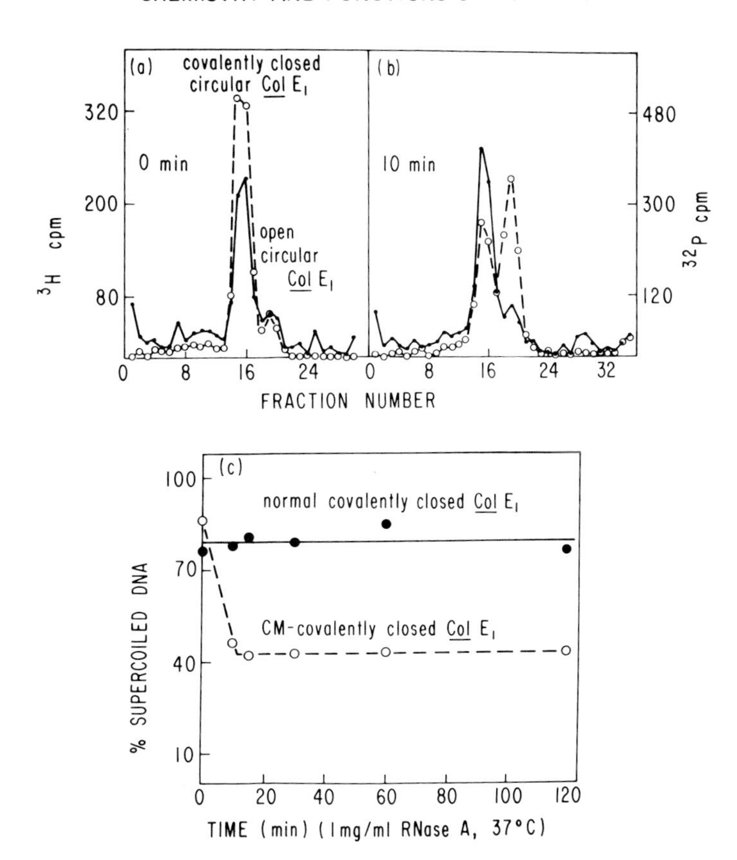

Figure 9 - Sensitivity of covalently-closed CM-$\underline{\text{Col}}E_1$ DNA to RNase A. Mixtures of supercoiled non-CM $\underline{\text{Col}}E_1$ and CM-$\underline{\text{Col}}E_1$ were incubated with RNase A for various time periods. Following RNase A treatment, the reaction mixture was analyzed on sucrose density gradients. (a) Incubation for 10 min at 37°C in the absence of RNase A; (b) incubation for 10 min at 37°C in the presence of RNase A; (c) relative amounts of the supercoiled DNA form of $\underline{\text{Col}}E_1$ DNA purified from chloramphenicol treated and untreated E. coli ($\underline{\text{Col}}E_1$) cells after incubation for various lengths of time with RNase A. The top of the sucrose density gradient is on the right in each case. (●——●) non-CM $\underline{\text{Col}}E_1$; (o----o) CM-$\underline{\text{Col}}E_1$. (From Blair et. al. (27)).

supercoiled DNA converts over 40% of the CM-*Col*E_1 DNA from a form sedimenting at the rate characteristic of an open circular molecule. Non-CM-*Col*E_1 DNA is not affected by the RNase treatment. Electron microscopy and alkaline sucrose gradient analyses of the isolated product of the RNase treatment of CM-*Col*E_1 supercoiled DNA clearly demonstrated that the conversion involves a supercoiled to open circular DNA transition with less than 3% of the product molecules in the linear form (27). Ribonuclease H, shown to be specific for the RNA portion of DNA-RNA hybrids, also induces the loss of the covalently-closed form of CM-*Col*E_1 DNA (27). Ribonuclease T_1 has no effect on CM-*Col*E_1 supercoiled DNA under the conditions employed. It is reasonable to conclude from these results that ribonucleotides are covalently integrated within the covalently-closed circular DNA structure of CM-*Col*E_1 DNA (27).

The number and strand specificity of RNase sensitive sites in the sensitive CM-*Col*E_1 DNA molecules were examined by centrifuging RNase-nicked CM-*Col*E_1 DNA through an alkaline sucrose gradient to separate the circular and linear strands followed by a strand specificity test on the separated strands utilizing the poly-(U,G) cesium chloride centrifugation method. The ratio of circular to linear strands in the alkaline sucrose gradient profile given in Figure 10 indicates that at least 80% of the open circular DNA product of RNase treatment contained only one nicked strand. The lack of a significant level of trailing from the peak of linear strands indicates that most of the nicked DNA strands possessed a single RNase sensitive site. The poly-(U,G) secium chloride gradient results (Figure 10) revealed that the circular and linear strands consisted of equal numbers of each of the complementary *Col*E_1 DNA strands. It is, thus, clear that the RNase sensitive site in the CM-*Col*E_1 DNA is distributed randomly between the two strands in the plasmid DNA.

It is possible that the RNase sensitivity of CM-*Col*E_1 DNA arises as an artifact of the exposure of

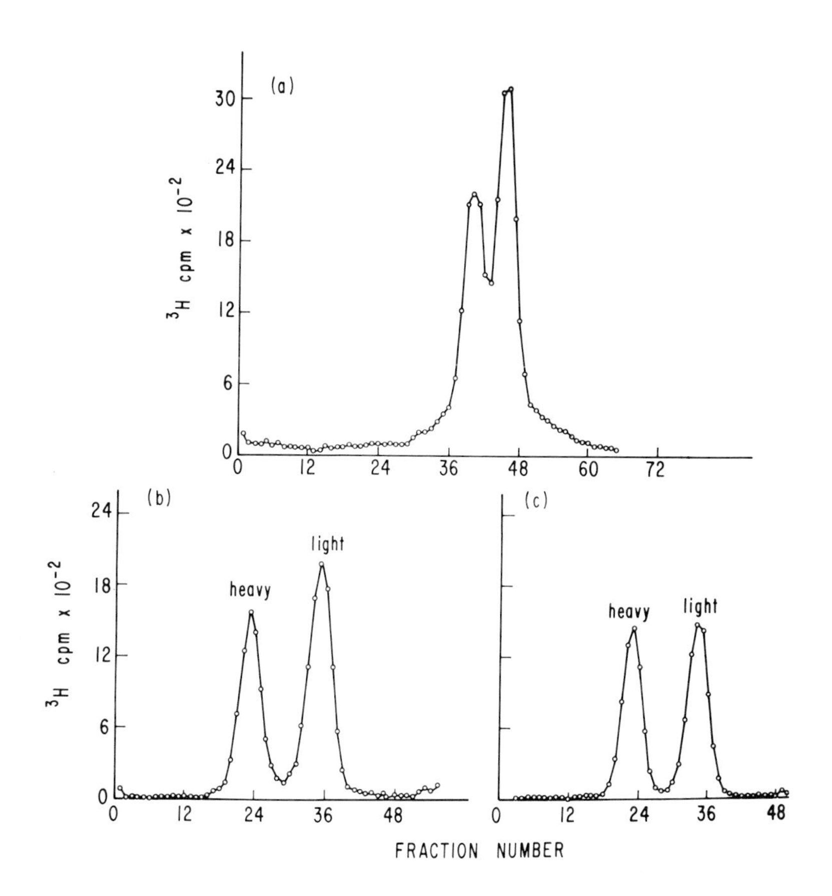

Figure 10 - Strand specificity of the RNase A sensitive site. After treatment of CM-ColE$_1$ DNA with RNase A, the open circular DNA product of the reaction was purified by dye-cesium chloride equilibrium centrifugation. The purified open circular ColE$_1$ DNA was layered on a 5-20% alkaline sucrose density gradient and centrifuged under conditions that separate the circular and linear single strands. The top of the alkaline sucrose density gradient (a) is on the right. Fractions of the faster (circular) peak and the slower (linear) peak were pooled separately and

(Figure 10, cont'd) analyzed on cesium chloride gradients containing poly-(U,G). (b) Poly-(U,G) cesium chloride equilibrium centrifugation of the material from the single stranded circular pool. (c) Poly-(U,G) cesium chloride equilibrium centrifugation of the material from the single stranded linear pool. (From Blair _et_. _al_. (27)).

colicinogenic cells to chloramphenicol, possibly as a result of the infrequent erroneous insertion of ribonucleotides during DNA polymerization. This explanation cannot be ruled out on the basis of the data presented at this time. On the other hand, the rifampicin sensitivity of _Col_E_1 DNA synthesis indicates an essential role for RNA in _Col_E_1 replication.

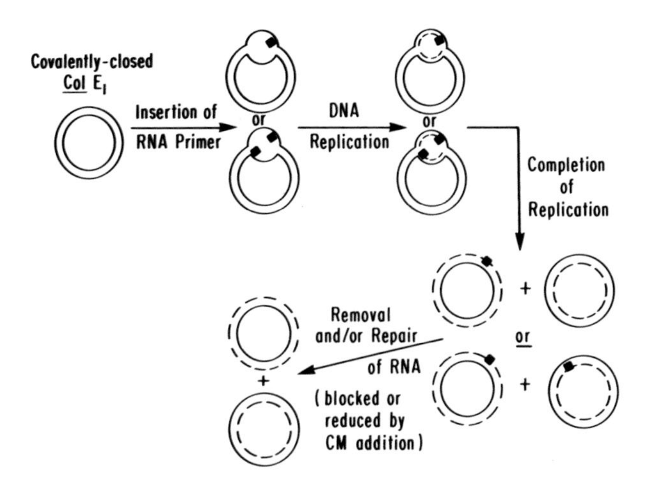

Figure 11 - Primer model for the formation of RNA-containing _Col_E_1 DNA. The initial steps of DNA synthesis involve the addition of deoxyribonucleotides to primer RNA that is complementary to a single site

(Figure 11, cont'd) on either DNA strand. Either a single RNA primer molecule, complementary to one or the other strand is involved in the duplication of any one circular DNA molecule, or synthesis proceeds bidirectionally from two primer RNA molecules present in a single replicating DNA molecule. Normally, the RNA primer is removed immediately before or after completion of replication of the circular DNA, however, in the presence of chlorampenicol RNA-containing, supercoiled $\underline{ColE}_1$ DNA molecules accumulate. (From Blair *et. al.* (27)).

Figure 11 illustrates a possible model for the formation of RNA-containing $\underline{ColE}_1$ supercoils as a result of a primer role that the RNA may be playing in the initiation of $ColE_1$ DNA synthesis. The randomness of the RNase sensitive site with respect to the two strands requires, according to this model, that either initiation of DNA synthesis is unidirectional and random with respect to the DNA strand, or synthesis is bidirectional and initiated with short RNA fragments from both strands of the replicating molecule.

In support of the physiological significance of the RNase sensitive CM-$\underline{ColE}_1$ DNA are the additional observations that the generation of these molecules in the presence of chloramphenicol requires active $\underline{ColE}_1$ DNA synthesis and is inhibited by the addition of rifampicin to the cells (27). It is of obvious importance at this time to determine the uniqueness and relative position of the RNase sites in the two plasmid DNA strands.

Concluding Remarks

Studies on the chemistry of colicinogenic factors have revealed several unique properties of circular DNA and complexes of circular DNA and protein. The message from these observations with respect to our detailed understanding of the biochemical events in the duplication and conjugal transfer of colicinogenic factors is not fully understood. Meanwhile, the great variety of plasmid elements continue to provide a rich source of diverse circular DNA molecules for a multi-faceted approach towards a genetic and biochemical understanding of the duplication and exchange of genetic material.

Acknowledgements

The studies described in this presentation were supported by U.S. Public Health Service research grant AI-07194, National Science Foundation research grant 6B-29492, and a U.S. Public Health Service Research Career Development Award (K04-6M07821).

References

1. J. Vinograd and J. Lebowitz, J. Gen. Physiol. 49, 103 (1966).
2. R. Radloff, W. Bauer and J. Vinograd, Proc. Nat. Acad. Sci. U.S.A. 57, 1514 (1967).
3. M. Bazaral and D.R. Helinski, J. Mol. Biol. 36, 185 (1968).
4. T.F. Roth and D.R. Helinski, Proc. Nat. Acad. Sci. U.S.A. 58, 650 (1967).
5. R.C. Clowes, X Int. Congr. Microbiol., Mexico, 1970, 58 (Cd-1).
6. F.T. Hickson, T.F. Roth and D.R. Helinski, Proc. Nat. Acad. Sci. U.S.A. 58, 1731 (1967).
7. D.B. Clewell and D.R. Helinski, Biochem. Biophys. Res. Commun. 41, 150 (1970).
8. D.B. Clewell and D.R. Helinski, Proc. Nat. Acad. Sci. U.S.A. 62, 1159 (1969).
9. J. Vinograd, J. Lebowitz, R. Radloff, R. Watson and P. Laipis, Proc. Nat. Acad. Sci. U.S.A. 53, 1104 (1965).
10. W. Goebel and D.R. Helinski, Proc. Nat. Acad. Sci. U.S.A. 61, 1406 (1968).
11. D.B. Clewell and D.R. Helinski, J. Bacteriol. 110, 1135 (1972).
12. D.R. Helinski and D.B. Clewell, Ann. Rev.

Biochem. 40, 899 (1971).
13. W. Gilbert and D. Dressler, Cold Spring Harbor Symp. Quant. Biol. 33, 473 (1968).
14. J. Inselburg and M. Fuke, Proc. Nat. Acad. Sci. U.S.A. 68, 2839 (1971).
15. D.B. Clewell and D.R. Helinski, Biochem. Biophys. Res. Commun. 40, 608 (1970).
16. D.B. Clewell and D.R. Helinski, Biochemistry 9, 4428 (1970).
17. D.G. Blair, D.B. Clewell, D.J. Sherratt and D.R. Helinski, Proc. Nat. Acad. Sci. U.S.A. 68, 210 (1971).
18. B.C. Kline and D.R. Helinski, Biochemistry 10, 4975 (1971).
19. W. Szybalski, H. Kubinski, Z. Hradecna and W.C. Summers, Meth. in Enzym., ed. L. Grossman and K. Moldave, (Acad. Press, New York, N.Y., 1971). Vol. XXI, Part D, pp. 383-413.
20. D. Vapnek and W.D. Rupp, J. Mol. Biol. 53, 287 (1970).
21. D.T. Kingsbury and D.R. Helinski, Biochem. Biophys. Res. Commun. 41, 1538 (1970).
22. D.B. Clewell, B. Evenchick and J.W. Cranston, Nature, New Biol. 237, 29 (1972).
23. D.R. Brutlag, R. Schekman and A. Kornberg, Proc. Nat. Acad. Sci. U.S.A. 68, 2826 (1971).
24. K.G. Lark, J. Mol. Biol. 64, 47 (1972).
25. B.C. Kline, Biochem. Biophys. Res. Commun. 46, 2019 (1972).
26. W. Wickner, D. Brutlag, R. Schekman and A. Kornberg, Proc. Nat. Acad. Sci. U.S.A. 69, 965 (1972).
27. D.G. Blair, D.J. Sherratt, D.B. Clewell and D.R. Helinski, Proc. Nat. Acad. Sci. U.S.A. 69, 2518 (1972).

CHEMISTRY OF COLICINS

Jordan Konisky

In recent years comparative studies of physiologically related proteins have contributed to an understanding of both evolutionary processes and structure-function relations (for a review, see 1). In this regard, comparative studies of the related bactericidal proteins, colicins, may lead to knowledge that is useful not only to workers interested in colicins, but to molecular biologists interested in general aspects of protein structure. It is the purpose of this talk to examine current information available concerning the structure of colicins.

In the past few years several colicins have been purified and characterized to such a degree that one can begin to ask questions concerning the possible correlations between the biological specificities exhibited by colicin molecules and their gross chemical and physical structure. My approach in discussing the chemistry of colicins will be to first describe in some detail the work which we have carried out concerning the characterization of the I-colicins. This will be followed by a discussion of the characterization of other colicins by other workers.

Table I summarizes the biochemical effects observed after treatment of sensitive *Escherichia coli* with each of the colicins under consideration. It is possible to group these colicins into three classes, according to their specific mode of action. Thus, treatment of sensitive *Escherichia coli* strains with colicin Ia (2), Ib (2), K (3), or E_1 leads to concomitant inhibition of all macromolecular synthesis. In addition, colicin K and E_1 have been shown to inhibit selective metabolic processes which are dependent upon electron transport such as active transport of potassium (3,4). Although the colicins included in this class inhibit the production of ATP (2,5), recent experiments with colicin E_1 (6) indicate that lowering of ATP levels may not be the primary lesion in colicin-treated cells. It has been

TABLE I

Biochemical Effects of Various Colicins on Sensitive Cells

Colicin	Ia	Ib	K	E1	E2	E3	D
Inhibition of:							
RNA Synthesis	+	+	+	+	(+)	-	-
DNA Synthesis	+	+	+	+	+	-	-
Protein Synthesis	+	+	+	+	(+)	+	+
DNA Degradation	-	-	-	-	+	-	
Specific Ribosome Inactivation	-	-	-	-	-	+	
Respiration	-	-	-	-	-	-	
ATP Production	+	+	+	+	-	-	
Active Transport of Potassium			+	+	-	-	
Phospholipid Synthesis	+	+	+				

suggested that each of the colicins in this class may be acting by interfering with energy supplying reactions located in the bacterial membrane. Unlike those colicins found in the first class, colicin E_2 has a specific effect on DNA, causing both the inhibition of DNA synthesis and DNA degradation (7). The third class is composed of colicins E_3 and D which specifically affect protein synthesis (3,8). Treatment of cells with colicin E_3 has been shown to result in ribosome inactivation (9), presumably by a specific cleavage of 16S ribosomal RNA (10).

Part I

I-colicins are classified by their activity spectrum on various strains of *E. coli*. Strain NO49/I (see Table II) is a mutant of strain *E. coli*

TABLE II

Colicin	Indicator Strain			
	NO49	NO49/I	NO49(Ia)	NO49(Ib)
Ia	s	r	imm	s
Ib	s	r	s	imm
E3	s	s	s	s

S, sensitive; r, resistant; imm, immune

TABLE III

Sensitivity of Colicin Ia to Various Agents

Addition	Activity	% Control
1. None	81	100
Trypsin	< 1	< 2.4
RNase	81	100
DNase	81	100
Heat (5 min at 100° C)	< 1	< 2.4
2. None	24	100
Phospholipase C	24	100
3. None	60	100
Subtilisin	< 1	< 1.7

K12 NO49 selected for resistance to colicin Ia. This mutant has simultaneously gained resistance to colicin Ib. Furthermore, it can be shown that NO49/I is defective in its ability to adsorb either colicin (2, Konisky and Cowell, manuscript in preparation). This finding suggests that these colicins adsorb to common bacterial receptors and, thus, by the classification scheme of Fredericq (11) are included in the colicin I class. However, the two colicins can be distinguished by their immunity specificities. Strain NO49 (Ia) which has the capacity to produce colicin Ia is not sensitive to low concentrations of colicin Ia, but is sensitive to colicin Ib, and *vice versa* (2,12). This particular kind of resistance towards homologous colicin is called *immunity*. Note that colicin E_3 is sensitive to all of the strains tested.

In view of their common biological properties, the I-colicins afford one an ideal system in which to study correlations between colicin structure and biological specificities. It is reasonable to suppose that colicins Ia and Ib have common amino acid sequences with regard to mode of action and receptor specificity, yet different amino acid sequences involved in immunity specificity. Thus comparative physical and chemical studies of these molecules may lead to information concerning the structural features involved in the immunity mechanism.

The sensitivity of crude colicin Ia to various agents is shown in Table III. Colicin activity is sensitive to proteolytic enzymes and heat, but refractory to nucleases and phospholipase C. These results are not surprising since other workers have shown that other colicins are protein (13). Furthermore, at a time when our studies were initiated, Herschmann and Helinski (14) had established that greater than 98% of the dry weight of purified colicins E_2 and E_3 was accounted for by their amino acid content.

Colicins Ia and Ib can be purified by standard methods used to purify proteins. Both colicins are purified to homogeneity with comparable yields by a

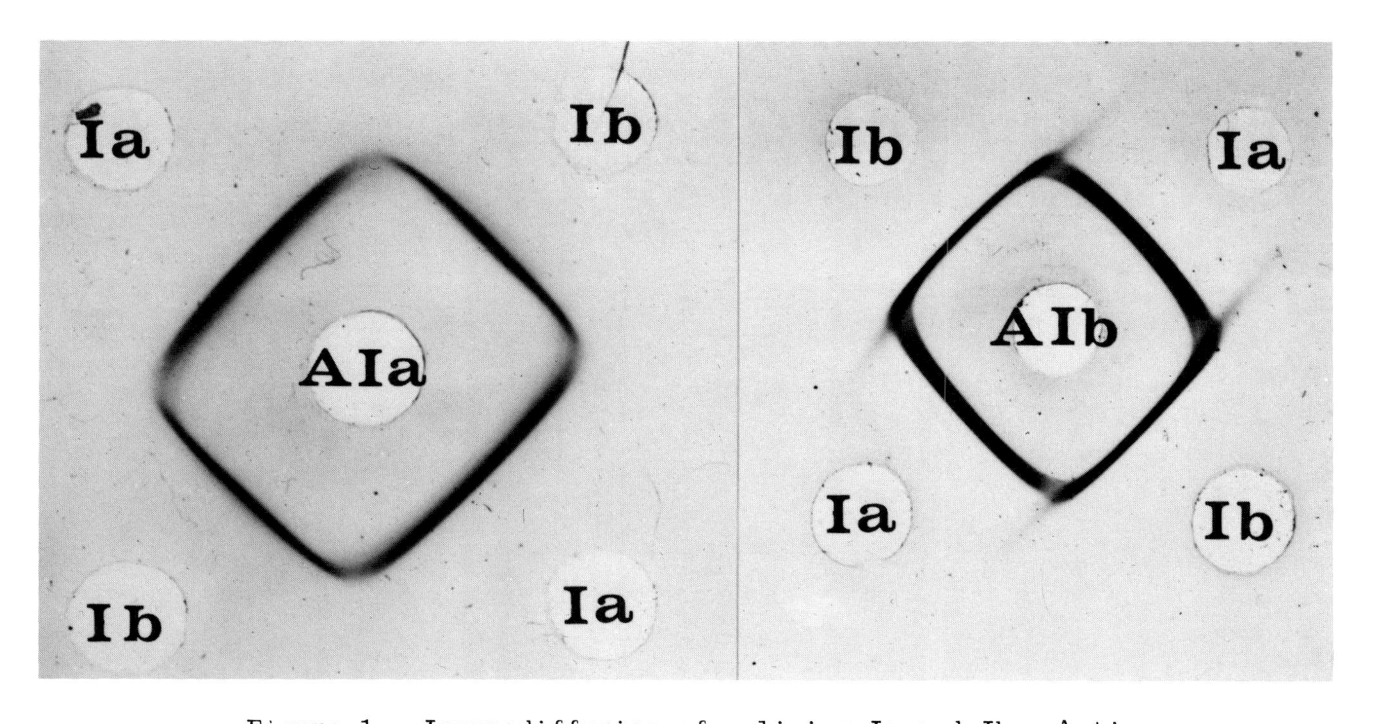

Figure 1 - Immunodiffusion of colicins Ia and Ib. Anti-colicin Ia or Ib gamma globulin was placed on the center well (AIa or AIb) and the purified colicin placed in peripheral wells (Ia or Ib).

TABLE IV

Amino Acid Compositions of Colicins Ia and Ib

Amino Acid	Colicin Ia Residues	Colicin Ib Residues
Lysine	69	60
Histidine	8	9
Arginine	49	50
Aspartic Acid	87	92
Threonine	50	33
Serine	44	30
Glutamic Acid	78	84
Proline	17	21
Glycine	43	38
Alanine	85	87
Valine	37	31
Methionine	5	8
Isoleucine	41	44
Leucine	60	59
Tyrosine	15	16
Phenylalanine	17	23
Tryptophane	7	8
TOTAL	712	693

common purification scheme (15) suggesting common physiochemical properties and perhaps structural features. That this is indeed the case can be demonstrated by immunological analysis on Ouchterlony double diffusion plates. Both purified colicins exhibit a single precipitin line with either homologous or heterologous anti-colicin gamma globulin (Figure 1).

In polyacrylamide gel electrophoresis at pH 8.6, colicins Ia and Ib migrate towards the cathode indicating that they have a basic isoelectric point (pI). This was confirmed by isoelectric focusing experiments in which it was found that colicin Ia and Ib have an isoelectric point of approximately 10 and 9.5, respectively (16).

Amino acid analyses revealed the residue frequencies shown in Table IV. The two colicins show a

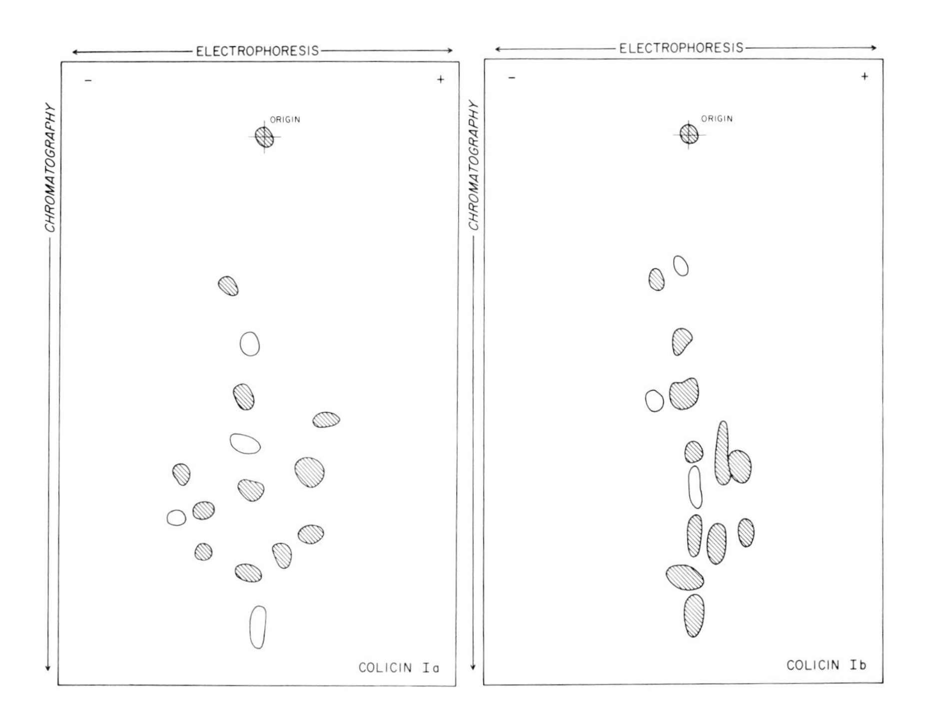

Figure 2 - Radioautograph of the peptide maps prepared from the tryptic digests of iodinated colicin Ia or Ib (16). Hatched spots are those of highest intensity.

similar amino acid composition. Both have a high content of basic amino acids and low amounts of hydrophobic groups. Neither colicin contained cysteine. The NH_2-terminal residue of colicin Ia and Ib was found to be serine.

That the similar amino acid compositions of colicin Ia and Ib reflect primary sequence homologies can be demonstrated by fingerprint analysis. Tryptic digestion yielded poorly resolved peptide maps due to the large lysine plus arginine content per colicin

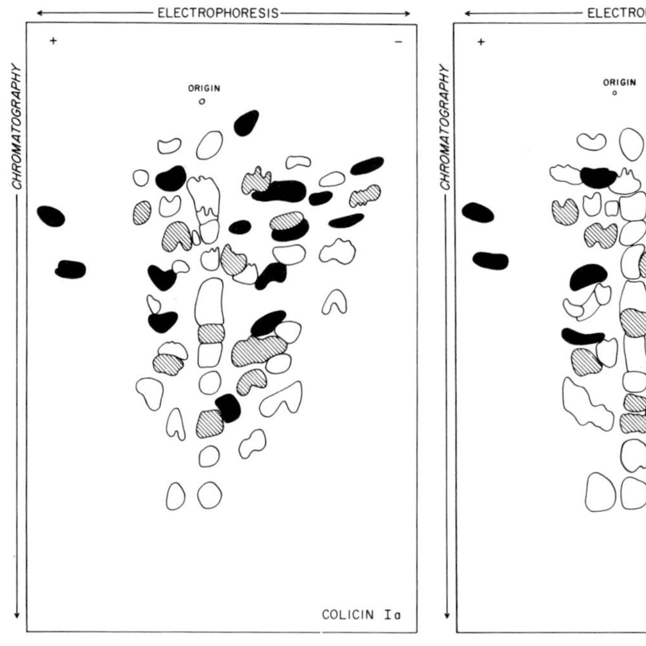

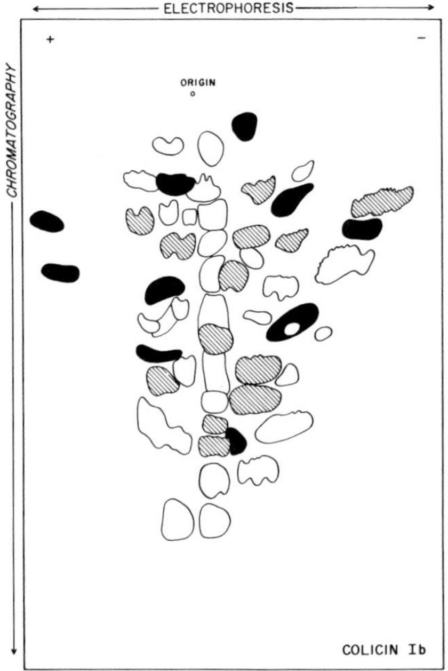

Figure 3 - Two dimensional peptide map of tryptic digest of colicin Ia and Ib (16). Spots with solid outline indicate arginine containing peptides (phenanthrenequinone positive). Hatched spots indicate arginine containing peptides of blue fluorescence under ultraviolet light. The other arginine peptides showed green to yellow fluorescence. Filled spots indicate well resolved ninhydrine positive but phenanthrenequinone negative peptides.

molecule (approximately 115 residues). Thus, selective procedures were used to localize specific classes of peptides. In the experiment shown in Figure 2, the colicins were iodinated with radioactive ^{125}iodine prior to trypsin digestion, and the iodine containing peptides (containing tryosine and/or histidine) were localized on fingerprint maps by autoradiography. Figure 3 shows tracings of experiments in which arginine containing peptides are specifically localized by reaction with phenanthrenequinone. In addition well resolved ninhydrin positive but non-

TABLE V

Physical Properties of Colicins Ia and Ib

Molecular Parameters	Colicin	
	Ia	Ib
Property		
$S^o_{20,w}$	3.57S	3.67S
$D^o_{20,w}$ (x 10^7 cm^2 sec^{-1})	4.12	4.32
$\bar{v}$ (milliliters per g)	0.733	0.736
Molecular Weight		
Equilibrium Centrifugation	75,000	80,800
Sedimentation-diffusion	78,800	78,100
SDS-acrylamide	79,000	80,000
$f/f_o = (f/f_o)_h\ (f/f_o)_a$	1.82	1.76
f/f_o (0.3g H_2O per g protein)	1.63	1.57
Axial Ratio		
Prolate	11	11
Oblate	14	14

arginine containing peptides are shown. From these experiments it was concluded that half of the iodinated peptides and greater than 80% of the arginyl peptides are identical, and therefore, that there exists extensive sequence homology between these two colicins (16).

Table V summarizes the physical properties of purified colicins Ia and Ib. Both colicins are of similar size and shape. The molecular weights as determined by sodium dodecyl sulfate acrylamide gel electrophoresis are identical to those obtained by hydrodynamic methods, indicating that both colicins consist of a single polypeptide chain of molecular weight 80,000. Data based on sedimentation velocity and diffusion measurements show f/f_o values of 1.82 and 1.76 for colicins Ia and Ib, respectively, where f is the determined frictional coefficient and f_o is the calculated frictional coefficient of an unhydrated sphere of molecular weight and partial specific volume equal to that of the particular colicin. Two explanations are commonly invoked to interpret discrepancies in the frictional coefficient obtained by these two methods: (1) the molecules may carry bound water, (2) the molecules may be elongated rather than spherical. These explanations are not mutually exclusive.

From the molecular weight (approximately 80,000) and partial specific volume (0.73 g per milliliter) of colicin Ia and Ib (15), one can calculate anhydrous volumes of 9.7×10^{-20} cm^3 per particle for the two colicins. For a spherical molecule this corresponds to a diameter of approximately 57 Angstroms. In order to be consistent with the hydrodynamic data, such a molecule would require approximately 3.5 g bound water per g of colicin. This would correspond to a ratio of 20 water molecules per amino acid residue which is impossibly high. On the other hand, assuming no hydration, the molecules can be considered anhydrous ellipsoids of revolution with an axial ratio of 16 and 21 for the prolate and oblate, respectively. Assuming 0.3 g water per g colicin which is considered a reasonable estimate for proteins (17), the colicins can be considered to have an axial ratio of 11 for the prolate and 14 for the oblate forms. For idealized ellipsoids of revolution, one can use this axial ratio to calculate dimensions for the prolate (minor axis, 25 Angstroms; major axis, 272 Angstroms) and for the oblate (minor axis, 10 Angstroms; major axis, 140 Angstroms). The preponderance of polar amino acids for the two colicins would be expected for rather extended molecules (18).

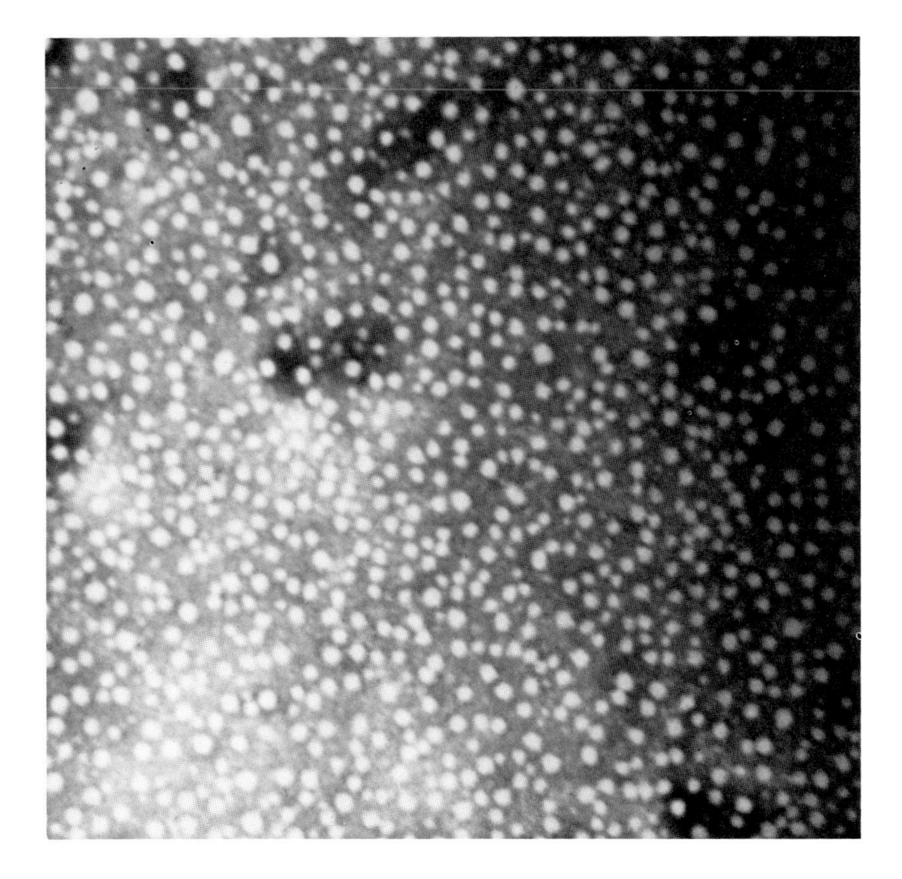

Figure 4 - Electron micrograph of purified colicin Ia. The colicin was negatively stained with 2% potassium phosphotungstate.

Figure 4 is an electron micrograph of negatively stained colicin Ia. Colicin Ia appears as a rounded structure having a diameter of approximately 210 Angstroms. Grids containing preparations of colicin preparation yielded a corresponding decrease in the number of particles seen per grid. Although we cannot unambiguously rule out distortion artifacts, the colicin does maintain full bacteriocidal activity in the phosphotungstate solution used for negative staining. As described above, anhydrous spherical molecules of these colicins would be expected to have a diameter of approximately 57 Angstroms. The larger diameter as demonstrated by negative staining would seem to rule out the possibility that our f/f_0 ratios are due to hydration effects. We feel that internal hydration is unlikely since tungstate can penetrate very small holes, and thus our molecules would have appeared "speckled" with stain or else obscured altogether (19). The electron micrographs show no evidence of prolate shaped molecules. On the other hand, they are consistent with oblate shaped structures. Although our hydrodynamic measurements predict a diameter 60-70 angstroms less than that observed, this calculation makes use of equations derived on the basis of idealized ellipsoids of revolution. The hydrodynamic formulae involved in the calculations may not be strictly applicable to protein molecules. Indeed, it has been demonstrated that calculations based on hydrodynamic data are not always borne out by electron microscopic data (18). Hence, although we favor an oblate "plate-like" structure for colicins Ia and Ib, the definitive shape of native colicins cannot be considered as established at this time.

Part II

Chemical and physical information is available for colicins E_1 (20), E_2 (14), E_3 (14), K (21), and D (22). Figure 5 shows the amino acid compositions of those colicins which inhibit all macromolecular synthesis. These colicins have characteristically

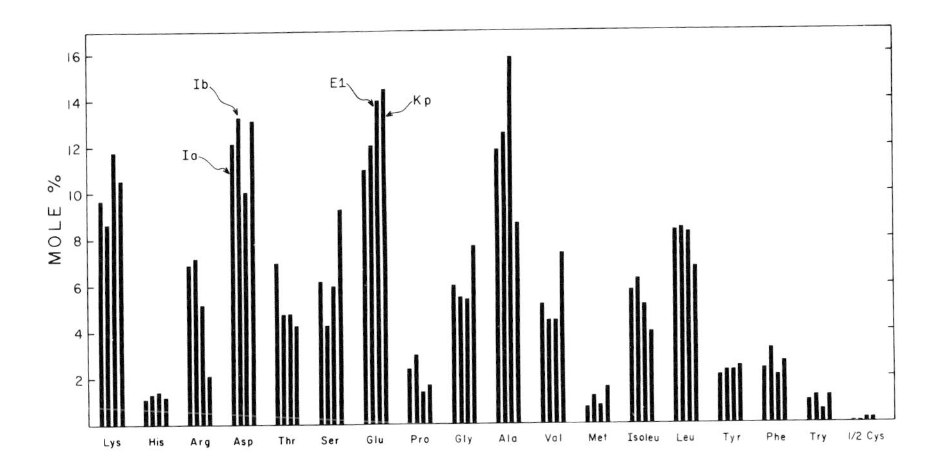

Figure 5 - Amino acid composition of colicins Ia, Ib, E_1 and K.

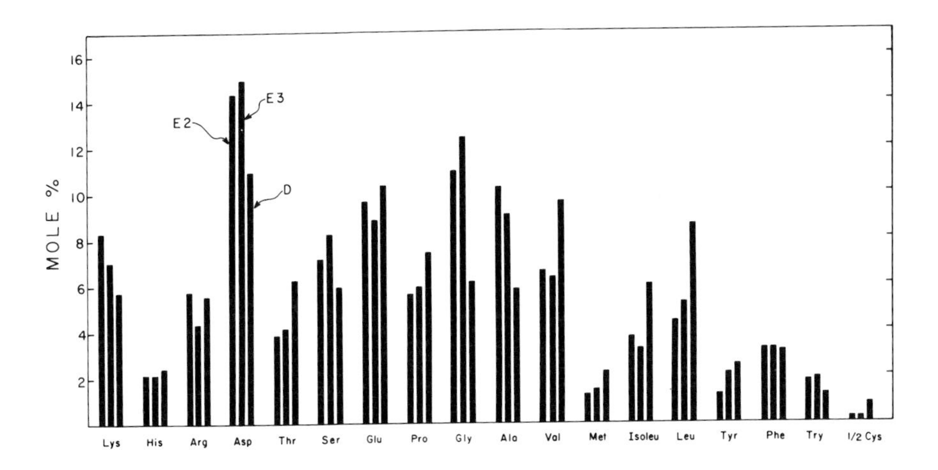

Figure 6 - Amino acid composition of colicins E_2, E_3 and D.

low contents of proline, glycine, methionine, and cysteine, and high amounts of lysine. The amino acid compositions of colicins E_2, E_3, and D are compared in Figure 6. It is clear that colicins E_2 and E_3 which have quite different modes of action are more

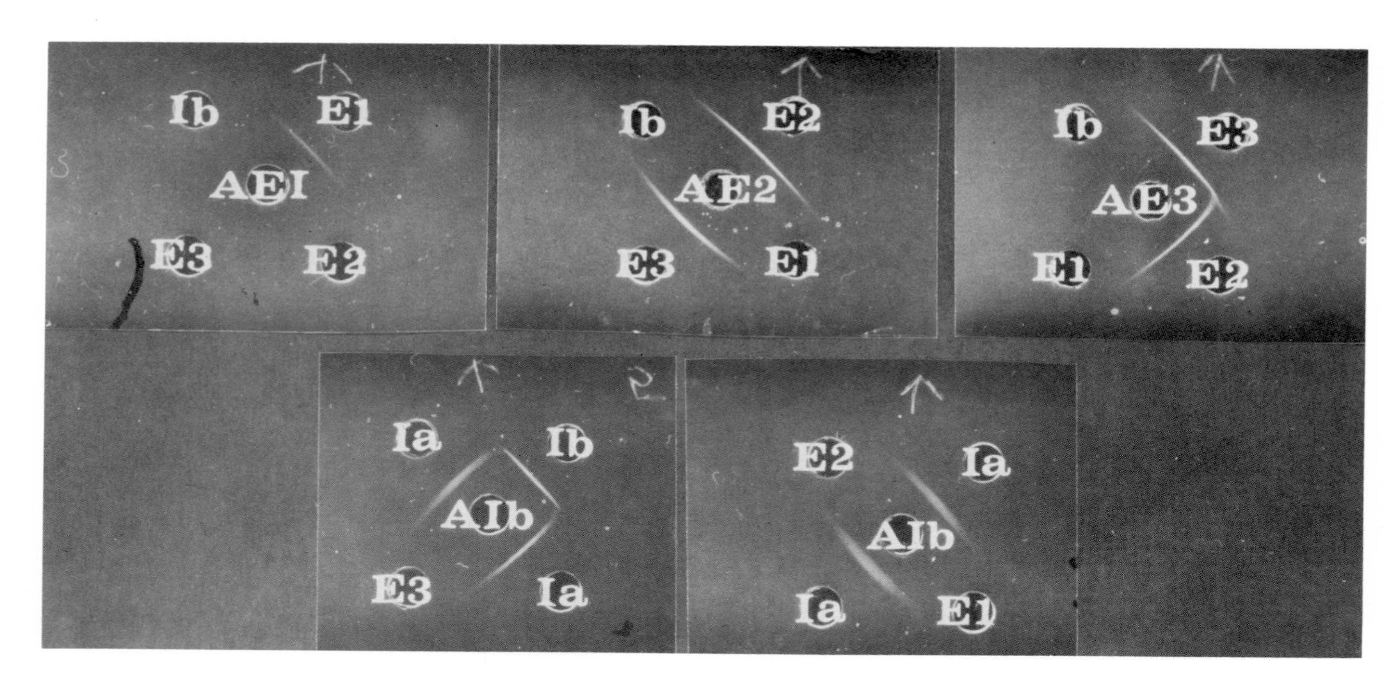

Figure 7 - Immunodiffusion of colicins Ia, Ib, E_1, E_2 and E_3. The indicated sera or purified gamma globulin was placed in the center well. Peripheral wells contained the indicated purified colicin.

closely related to each other than is colicin E_3 to colicin D.

That colicins sharing similar modes of action are not necessarily structurally related is confirmed by immunological studies (Figure 7). Thus, Ouchterlony double diffusion analysis shows that colicin E_1 does not cross react with any of the colicins tested. However, as previously shown (14), colicins E_2 and E_3 share common antigenic specificities as do colicins Ia and Ib (23). Colicin K does not react with any of the sera described in Figure 7 (data not shown). It has been reported that colicin D is antigenically distinct from colicin E_3 (22).

Table VI summarizes the physical properties of the colicins under consideration. The colicins exhibit a range of molecular weights (45-89,000). Interestingly enough, those colicins which inhibit all macromolecular synthesis have characteristically high f/f_0 values. Thus colicins E_1 and K can be considered as either prolate shaped molecules with axial ratios of 15 and 10, respectively, or oblate shaped molecules with axial ratios 20 and 12 respectively.

TABLE VI

Physical Properties of Some Colicins

Molecular Parameters	Colicin					
	E1	K_p	K_c	E2	E3	D
Molecular Weight	63,000	45,000	69,000	62,000	60,000	89,000
S	3.0	2.86		4,0	4.1	4.41
$D_{20,w}$ (x 10^7 cm^2 sec^{-1})	4.2					
$\bar{v}$	0.725	0.71		0.725	0.725	0.74
$f/f_0 = (f/f_0)_h \cdot (f/f_0)_a$	2.02	1.70		1.45	1.40	1.58
f/f_0 (0.3g H_2O per g protein)	1.79	1.52		1.29	1.25	1.41
Axial Ratio						
Prolate	15	9.6		5.6	4.9	7.5
Oblate	20	11.8		6.2	5.5	8.8
pI	9.05	5.14, 5.21	5.7	7.63, 7.41	6.64	4.70

Colicins E_2, E_3 and D also have hydrodynamic properties indicative of axial asymmetry. However, their axial ratios for prolate or oblate shapes are not as extreme as for those colicins previously mentioned (see Table V).

Finally, Table V includes the isoelectric points (pI) of the various colicins.

Conclusions

(1) The purification and characterization of various colicins isolated from induced colicinogenic strains has convincingly established that colicins can exist as simple proteins.

(2) The common biological properties of colicins Ia and Ib are reflected in common structural features.

(3) In general there is little correlation between the mode of action of colicins and gross amino acid composition or antigenic properties. This is not surprising since mode of action is but one of several specificities found in colicin molecules. There does seem to be some suggestion of a correlation between receptor specificity and colicin structure. Thus, colicins E_2 and E_3 which are structurally related adsorb to a common receptor (24) which is distinct from El receptor (25). As stated above colicins Ia and Ib also adsorb to a common receptor.

(4) Colicins are elongated molecules. Those colicins which cause an inhibition of all macromolecular synthesis exhibit the highest degree of elongation.

(5) Colicins Ia and Ib appear to be oblate (plate-like) molecules.

Acknowledgment

Early work on the characterization of colicins Ia and Ib was carried out while the author served as a postdoctoral fellow in the laboratory of F. M. Richards, Yale University. The author thanks M. Nomura for gifts of purified colicins E_2, E_3 and K;

and D. Helinski for purified colicin E_1, and colicin E_1, E_2 and E_3 antisera. The author is grateful to R. E. Isaacson for carrying out the electron microscopic examination of colicin Ia and to B. S. Cowell for technical assistance. Work carried out in the author's laboratory was supported by United States Public Health Service Research Grant AI-10106.

References

1. Nolan, C. and Margoliash, E., Ann. Rev. Biochem., 37, 727 (1968).
2. Levisohn, R., Konisky, J., and Nomura, M., J. Bacteriol., 96, 811 (1968).
3. Nomura, M., and Maeda, A., Zentr. Bakteriol. Parasitenk, Abt. I. Orig., 196, 216 (1965).
4. Luria, S. E., Ann. Inst. Pasteur, 107, 67 (1964).
5. Fields, K. L., and Luria, S. E., J. Bacteriol., 97, 57 (1969).
6. Feingold, D. S., J. Membrane Biol., 3, 372 (1970).
7. Nomura, M., Cold Spring Harbor Symp. Quant. Biol., 28, 315 (1963).
8. Timmis, K., and Hedges, A. J., Biochim. Biophys. Acta, 262, 200 (1972).
9. Konisky, J. and Nomura, M., J. Mol. Biol., 26, 181 (1967).
10. Bowman, C. M., Dahlberg, J. E., Ikemura, T., Konisky, J., and Nomura, M., Proc. Natl. Acad. Sci., U.S., 68, 964 (1971).
11. Fredericq, P., Rev. Belge. Pathol. Med. Exp., 29, 1 (1948).
12. Stocker, B. A. D., Heredity, 21, 166 (1966).
13. Nomura, M., Ann. Rev. Microbiol., 21, 257 (1967).
14. Herschman, H. R., and Helinski, D. R., J. Biol. Chem., 242, 5360 (1967).
15. Konisky, J. and Richards, F. M., J. Biol. Chem., 245, 2972 (1970).
16. Konisky, J., J. Biol. Chem., In Press.
17. Cohn, E. J. and Edsall, J. T., In Proteins, Amino Acids, and Peptides, Rheinhold Publishing

Company, New York, P. 434 (1943).

18. Fisher, H. F., Proc. Natl. Acad. Sci., U.S., 51, 1285 (1964).
19. Valentine, R. C., Nature, Lond., 184, 1838 (1959).
20. Schwartz, S. A., and Helinski, D. R., J. Biol. Chem., 246, 6318 (1971).
21. Jesaitis, M. A., J. Exptl. Med., 131, 1016 (1970).
22. Timmis, K., J. Bacteriol., 109, 12 (1972).
23. Isaacson, R. E., and Konisky, J., J. Bacteriol., 109, 1322 (1972).
24. Maeda, A., and Nomura, M., J. Bacteriol., 91, 685 (1966).
25. Hill, C., and Holland, I. B., Bacteriol., 94, 677 (1967).

CHEMISTRY OF THE COLICIN E RECEPTOR

Sohair F. Sabet[1] and Carl A. Schnaitman

Introduction

Properties of the Envelope of Escherichia coli

In order to discuss the chemistry of colicin receptors, it is necessary to review first the structure and chemistry of the cell envelope on which these receptors are localized.

When cells of *E. coli* are fixed, embedded, and sectioned and examined in the electron microscope (Fig. 1) several distinct layers can be seen. There are two membranes surrounding the cell, the inner or cytoplasmic membrane and the outer membrane. These have an identical appearance with the exception that in intact cells a finely beaded layer is visible on the inner surface of the outer membrane. This beaded layer is lost on conversion of the cells to spheroplasts, and a number of studies have shown that this layer represents the rigid murein or peptidoglycan layer which is only a single molecule thick. The lipopolysaccharide which forms the actual outer surface of the cell is not visible in conventional micrographs such as Fig. 1, since the carbohydrate side chains do not take up heavy metal stains. However, when such preparations are stained with ferritin-coupled antibody directed against the O antigenic determinants on the lipopolysaccharide side chains it can be seen that the side chains extend quite far out from the surface of the outer membrane (1).

Figure 2 shows a schematic model of the *E. coli*

---

[1]Present Address: Department of Biology, Massachusetts Institute of Technology, Cambridge, Mass. 02139.

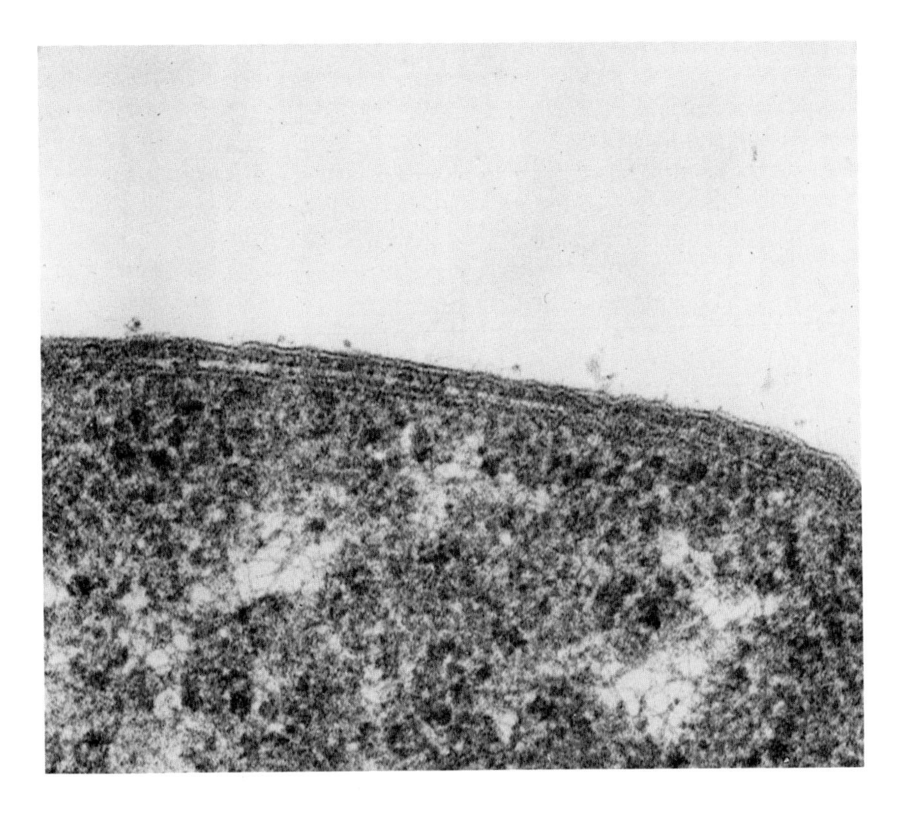

Figure 1 - Electron micrograph of a section of an *E. coli* cell showing the outer membrane, cytoplasmic membrane, and intervening peptidoglycan layer. 160,000 X.

envelope which is somewhat more detailed than the model which Dr. Luria presented earlier in this Symposium. This model is based on observations made in our laboratory and in a number of other laboratories over the last few years (2). Both the outer membrane and the cytoplasmic membrane contain phospholipid and protein, presumably in the form of bilayers. About half of the phospholipid of the envelope is found in the outer membrane, and about half in the cytoplasmic membrane. Recent studies indicate that the lipid composition is similar in both membranes (3). The protein composition of the two membranes is quite

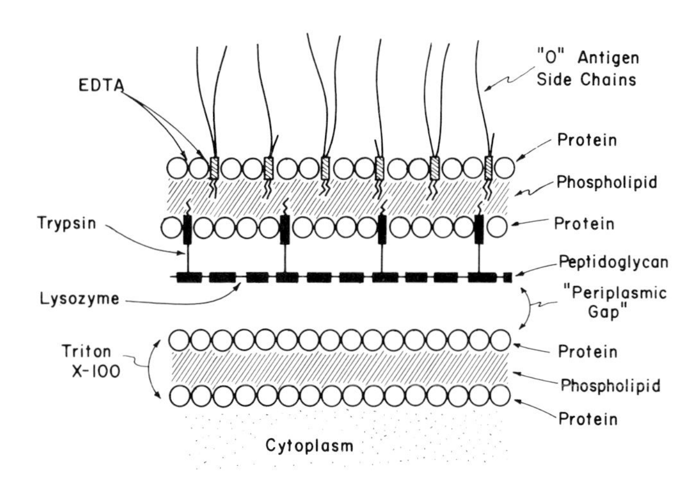

Figure 2 - Schematic representation of the envelope of E. coli. For simplicity the outer membrane are shown as simple bilayers. Arrows indicate the site of action of EDTA in the release of proteins and lipopolysaccharide from the outer membrane, and the action of trypsin in cleavage of the murein lipoprotein (6). Reproduced from Reference 2 with the permission of the Journal of Bacteriology.

different, both quantitatively and qualitatively. The outer membrane contains about two-thirds of the total protein of the envelope, and hence the outer membrane has a much lower ratio of lipid to protein.

In the presence of small amounts of divalent cations the solubility of the proteins of the two membranes is quite different, and this property is useful in separating and fractionating these membranes. If a crude envelope preparation from E. coli is extracted with the non-ionic detergent Triton X-100 in the absence of chelating agents to remove bound cations or in the presence of low levels of Mg^{++} only the proteins of the cytoplasmic membrane are solubilized (4). Even though such extraction removes much of the lipopolysaccharide and phospholipid of the outer membrane, the outer membrane and attached peptidoglycan layer retain their characteristic morphology. If the Triton-insoluble fraction (outer membrane plus peptidoglycan) is then re-extracted with Triton X-100 in the presence of EDTA about half of the protein of the outer membrane can then be solubilized (2).

Two other features of the model shown in Fig. 2 should be noted. First, the lipopolysaccharide is attached to the outer membrane, presumably by insertion of the lipid portion of this molecule into the lipid or hydrophobic layer of the outer membrane. Divalent cations must also be important in maintaining the attachment of lipopolysaccharide to the outer membrane, since EDTA causes release of lipopolysaccharide both from intact cells (5) and from isolated cell walls (2). A second feature is the presence of a small protein which contains covalently-bound lipid and which is covalently linked to the peptidoglycan. This protein has been extensively characterized by Braun and his associates (6,7,8) and probably functions as a "glue" holding the peptidoglycan layer to the outer membrane. By rough estimates this protein appears to account for about 10 per cent of the total protein of the outer membrane.

Figure 3 shows a comparison of the polypeptide patterns of the outer membrane and cytoplasmic membrane by polyacrylamide gel electrophoresis in the presence of SDS. In this case, the proteins of the two membranes were separated by Triton X-100 extraction. The cytoplasmic membrane contains polypeptides of a wide variety of sizes, and in good gels as many as 30 distinct bands can be identified. There are no major polypeptides in the cytoplasmic membrane. On the other hand, the outer membrane protein yields a much simpler pattern. Only seven or eight distinct bands are visible, and the bulk of the protein (about 70 per cent of the total) is present as a single major band with an apparent molecular weight of about 42,000.

The apparent simplicity of the polypeptide

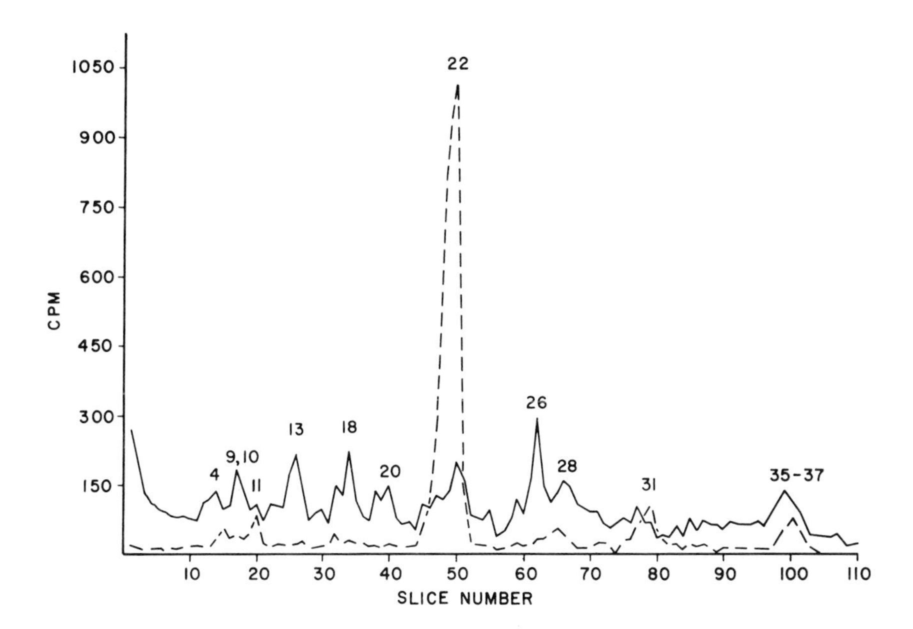

Figure 3 - Polypeptide profiles of ^{3}H-labeled cytoplasmic membrane protein (solid line) and ^{14}C-labeled cell wall protein (dashed line) on SDS polyacrylamide gel electrophoresis. In this and all succeeding gel profiles the top of the gel is to the left. In this experiment the cell wall and cytoplasmic membrane were separated by extraction with Triton X-100, and the samples were prepared for electrophoresis by dissolution in acidified dimethyl formamide, gel filtration on Sephadex LH-20 to remove lipid and Triton, and dialysis into SDS solution. Reproduced from Reference 4 with the permission of the Journal of Bacteriology.

profile is somewhat misleading, and since the polypeptide peak with an apparent molecular weight of 42,000 d. is the main contamination of the purified colicin receptor fraction it is worth commenting further on the problems associated with the major polypeptides of the outer membrane. The outer membrane polypeptide profile shown in Fig. 3 is obtained only when the outer membrane protein has been prepared for gel electrophoresis by one of two methods: Either by exposure of the protein to helix-promoting solvents such as acidified dimethyl formamide or 2-chloroethanol prior to exposure of the protein to SDS (as is the case in Fig. 3), or by dissolving the protein in excess SDS (about 2 mg SDS per mg protein) followed by boiling for 5 min or longer. In the latter case, addition of 8 M urea prior to boiling provides a somewhat sharper polypeptide profile, although this is not essential. If the outer membrane is simply dissolved in SDS at room temperature and applied to the gels, or is dissolved in SDS and heated to a temperature of less than 100^{0} C, a very complicated polypeptide pattern is obtained which does not resemble that which is shown in Fig. 3. This has led to considerable confusion in the literature concerning the true nature and number of polypeptides in the outer membrane or in crude envelope fractions (which contain primarily the outer membrane protein).

The reasons behind this rather confusing behavior of the outer membrane polypeptides are now becoming apparent on the basis of studies carried out by Bragg and Hou (9) and in our laboratory (C. Schnaitman, manuscript in preparation). Our studies of the cyanogen bromide peptides obtained from this 42,000 d. protein peak indicated the presence of at least three distinct polypeptides, all of which have an identical molecular weight of about 42,000 d. Bragg and Hou (9) showed that when preparations of the outer membrane which had been boiled in SDS solution were subjected to electrophoresis in SDS gels at pH 11.4 three distinct polypeptide bands could be resolved. Of these three polypeptides, two form higher molecular weight aggregates which are quite stable and can be dissociated to the 42,000 d. form only by boiling in SDS or by treatment with organic solvents. The third polypeptide exhibits an apparent molecular weight of less than 42,000 d. until it is either boiled in SDS solution or treated with an organic solvent, presumably due to some conformational change.

Preliminary Characterization of the Colicin E_3 Receptor

In order to attempt to solubilize and purify the colicin E_3 receptor, it was necessary to develop convenient assays for receptor activity. We have utilized two different types of assays. Both are "protection" assays based on the fact that the colicin is so strongly bound to the receptor that it is for all practical purposes irreversible. The first of these assays (Fig. 4) involves adding various amounts of colicin E_3 to a fixed, known amount of cells, incubating for a fixed time period, and then plating the mixture to determine the number of survivors. The same procedure is then followed with an identical sample of colicin which has been preincubated with a sample to be tested for receptor activity. Since the inactivation follows single-hit kinetics the 37 per cent survival point indicates that at that colicin concentration there is one killing unit of colicin present per cell. By determining the amount of additional colicin which must be added to reach the 37 per cent survival point in the presence of the receptor sample it is possible to calculate the number of killing units of colicin which have been bound to the receptor sample. This assay is relatively accurate, but it is time-consuming and involves a large number of platings.

The data shown in Fig. 4 represent one of our early experiments to determine the localization of the colicin E_3 receptor activity. In this experiment, cells of both colicin-sensitive and colicin-resistant strains were broken with a French press and the particulate fraction of the cells was separated into cell wall-enriched and cytoplasmic membrane-enriched fractions by centrifugation in a continuous sucrose gradient. Identical amounts of these envelope subfractions and of the original envelope preparations were then tested for receptor activity. The resistant strain showed no receptor activity in either the whole envelope or the sub-fractions. Receptor activity was present in both the cell wall and cytoplasmic membrane-enriched subfractions from the colicin-sensitive strains, but the bulk of the activity was in the cell wall-enriched fraction and the amount of receptor activity in the cytoplasmic membrane-enriched fraction was comparable to the amount of cell wall contamination present in the cytoplasmic membrane fraction. Hence the receptor seems to be present on the cell wall but not the cytoplasmic membrane.

In most of our experiments it was much more convenient to use a spot test for receptor activity. In this assay (not illustrated) a sample of colicin was diluted serially and a small sample of each serial dilution was then spotted on a plate containing a soft agar overlay seeded with a sensitive indicator strain. The end point is the highest dilution of the colicin which produces a clear spot. A sample to be tested for receptor activity was then preincubated with an identical amount of colicin, and diluted and plated in the same way. The receptor titer is then indicated by the shift in end point

TABLE I

Solubilization of Colicin E_3 Receptor Activity From Envelope Fraction of E. Coli C600 104

Test Material	% of Envelope Protein	Receptor Titer
Unfractionated Envelope	100%	10^3
Triton-soluble Fraction	36%	10^2
Triton-EDTA soluble Fraction (from Triton-insoluble wall)	18%	10^3
Triton-EDTA insoluble Fraction (from Triton-insoluble wall)	46%	10^1

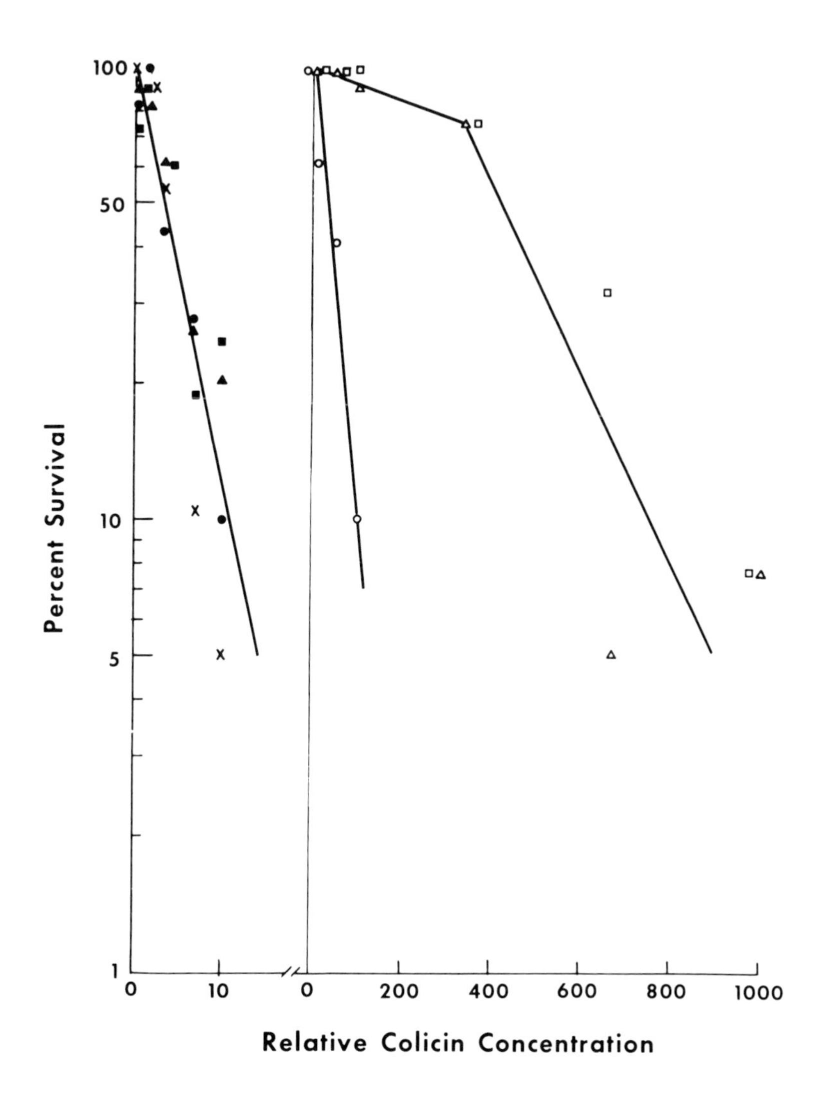

Figure 4 - An example of the survival curve method for the assay of colicin receptor activity. This experiment shows the protection of an indicator strain against killing by colicin E_3 by various envelope subfractions isolated from sensitive and resistant E. coli strains. Samples of the various subfractions were mixed with identical samples of

(Figure 4, con'd) various colicin dilutions, incubated, and then added to samples of a culture of the indicator strain. After a second incubation the indicator strain was plated and the number of survivors was determined. Envelope subfractions from the colicin-sensitive strain are as follows: Unfractionated envelope (open triangles), cell wall fraction (open squares), and cytoplasmic membrane fraction (open circles). Envelope subfractions from a colicin-resistant mutant are as follows: Unfractionated envelope (closed triangles), cell wall fraction (closed squares), and cytoplasmic membrane fraction (closed circles). The "X" indicates a control containing only colicin diluent in place of the envelope subfractions. Reproduced from Reference 10 with the permission of the Journal of Bacteriology.

to lower dilutions. In some of the initial experiments (10) ten-fold dilutions were used, but in later experiments two-fold dilutions were used for greater accuracy. This assay was particularly useful for locating receptor activity in fractions from chromatography.

The experiment shown in Table I was done using the spot assay, and provides further evidence that the colicin E_3 receptor is localized in the outer membrane. Only a small fraction of the receptor activity is solubilized when the crude envelope fraction is extracted with Triton X-100, a procedure which completely solubilizes the cytoplasmic membrane. We have since repeated this type of experiment by adding a small amount of Mg^{++} to the envelope prior to the Triton X-100 extraction, and this reduces the amount of receptor activity in the Triton-soluble fraction to zero. Low levels of Mg^{++} do not affect the solubility of the cytoplasmic membrane in Triton X-100 solution (4).

Table I also shows that the bulk of the receptor activity present in the Triton-insoluble cell wall fraction can be solubilized by re-extraction with Triton X-100 in the presence of EDTA. Since this appeared to be a good starting material for further purification of the receptor activity, the properties of this solubilized fraction were examined in greater detail.

The receptor activity present in the Triton-EDTA solubilized fraction exhibited the same specificity as the intact cell, and thus is unlikely to be due to some non-specific inactivation of the colicin. This is shown in Table II, since strains which were resistant to colicin E_3 but not to colicin K had no receptor activity for colicin E_3 in the Triton-EDTA soluble fraction, while this fraction did still contain receptor activity for colicin K. Similar results were obtained with strains specifically resistant for colicin K (10). Tolerant mutants which were

TABLE II

Comparison of Various E. Coli Strains with Respect to Colicin Sensitivity and Presence of Colicin Receptor Activity

E. coli Strain	Colicin Sensitivity:		Colicin Receptor Titer in Triton EDTA Soluble Fractions	
	Colicin E_3	Colicin K	Colicin E_3	Colicin K
K-12 X 478	+	+	10^3	---
K-12 Hfr	+	+	10^3	---
K-12 C600 104	+	+	10^3	10^2
K-12 C600 R/E_3	-	+	0	10^2
M1	-	-	0	---
B	-	+	0	10^2

still able to bind colicins had receptor activity in the Triton-EDTA soluble fraction (10).

Preliminary chemical experiments on the Triton-EDTA soluble fraction suggested that both protein and carbohydrate were required for receptor activity, since the activity was destroyed both by trypsin and by periodate oxidation. The receptor activity was fairly heat-stable, and could be precipitated with ammonium sulfate or ethanol without loss of activity (10). Ethanol precipitation has proved particularly useful during the purification of receptor activity, since it permits removal of the Triton X-100 which causes some problems with chemical determinations and with SDS gel electrophoresis. The Triton-EDTA solubilized material is evidently still aggregated, since it is partially excluded from Biogel A5M.

Purification of the Colicin E_3 Receptor

The general fractionation scheme for the purification of colicin E_3 receptor activity is shown in Figure 5. With this purification procedure it has been possible to enrich the colicin receptor activity several hundred fold with respect to the protein content of the crude envelope fraction.

Preliminary examination of a partially purified receptor fraction by SDS polyacrylamide gel electrophoresis indicated that a protein which migrated more slowly on the gels than the major cell wall polypeptide peak was enriched during the purification. This protein could not be detected in Triton-EDTA solubilized starting material. In order to demonstrate that this protein was in fact a specific component of the colicin E_3 receptor, the following experiment was done. A culture of a mutant specifically resistant to group E colicins (10) was grown on medium containing ^{14}C-labeled amino acids and an identical culture of the colicin-sensitive parent strain was grown on medium containing ^{3}H-labeled amino acids. The two cultures were mixed after harvesting, and were broken and fractionated together by the scheme shown in Figure 5. At various stages of purification the fractions were examined for their ^{14}C and ^{3}H protein patterns by SDS polyacrylamide gel electrophoresis. The crude envelope fraction and the Triton-EDTA soluble fraction (Figs. 6 and 7) gave protein patterns which were quite similar for ^{14}C and ^{3}H, and there was no

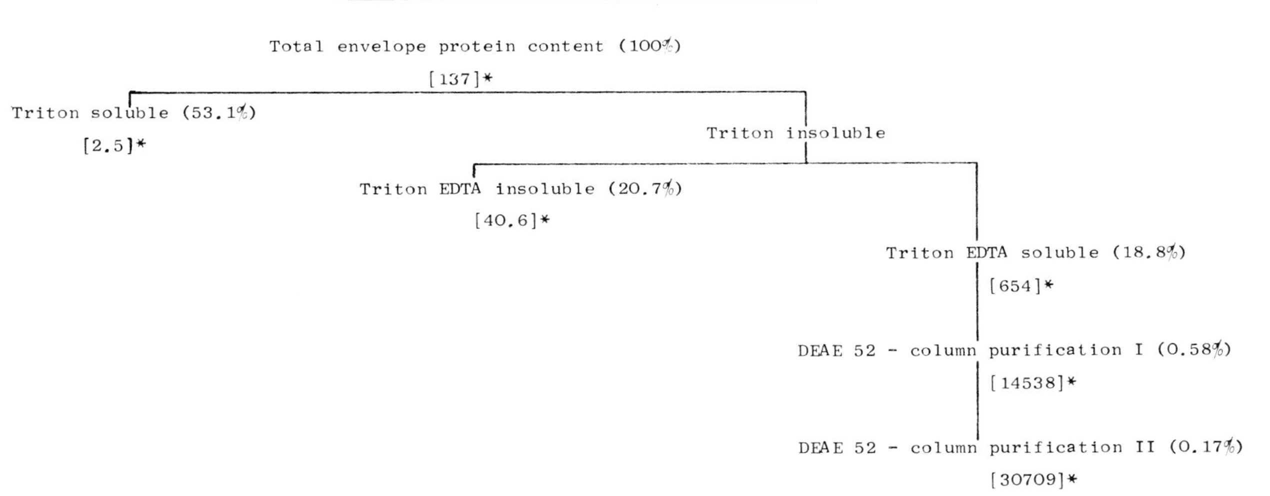

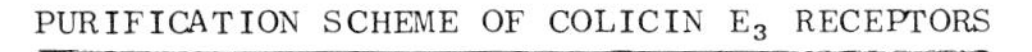

Figure 5 - Purification Scheme of Colicin E_3 Receptors. This figure illustrates the general scheme for the isolation and purification of colicin E_3 receptor activity (11), and shows a typical experiment. The numbers in parenthesis indicate the protein recovered in each fraction in terms of the percentage of the total envelope protein. The numbers in brackets indicate the specific activity of the colicin receptor in arbitrary units per mg protein.

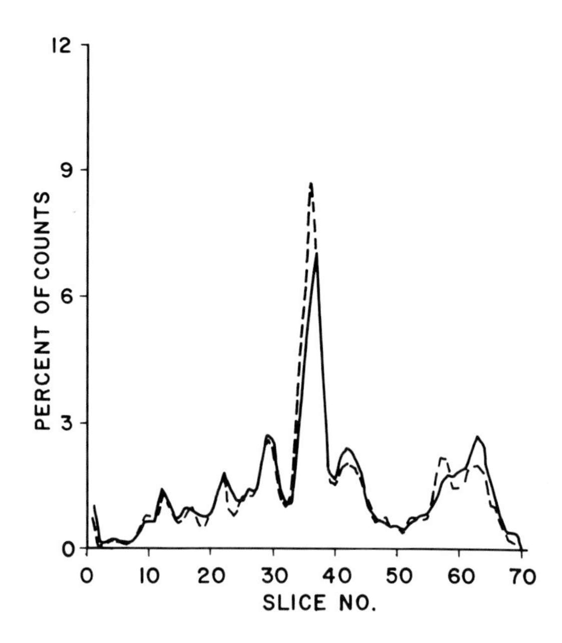

Figure 6 - SDS gel electrophoresis pattern of the crude envelope preparation isolated from a mixture of colicin-sensitive cells labeled with ^{3}H amino acids and colicin-resistant cells labeled with ^{14}C amino acids. The top of the gel is to the left, and to facilitate comparison the results are expressed as the percent of the total counts recovered from the gel for each isotope. The solid line indicates ^{3}H counts and the dashed line indicates ^{14}C counts. The sample was prepared for electrophoresis by dissolving in excess SDS solution, making the solution 8 M in urea, and boiling for 5 minutes. Reproduced from Reference 11 with the permission of the Journal of Biological Chemistry.

evidence at these stages of purification of any protein which was labeled only with ^{3}H. Figure 8 shows the first chromatography step of the Triton-EDTA soluble fraction on DEAE cellulose (DEAE column I). The

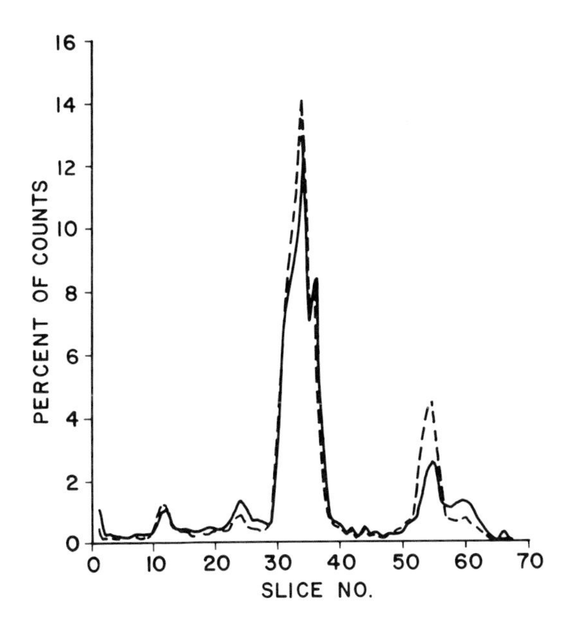

Figure 7 - SDS gel electrophoresis pattern of the Triton-EDTA soluble fraction from the mixed culture shown in Fig. 6. The solid line represents ^3H counts from the sensitive strain and the dashed line represents ^{14}C counts from the resistant strain. Conditions are as in Fig. 6. Note that there are only slight differences in the patterns of the two isotopes. Reproduced from Reference 11 with the permission of the Journal of Biological Chemistry.

bulk of the protein eluted at a low NaCl concentration, and this fraction contained no receptor activity. The colicin receptor activity eluted as a broad peak beginning at about 0.25 M NaCl. Since little protein eluted at this salt concentration there was a substantial purification of the receptor activity -- in some experiments a purification of 33-fold has been obtained with this chromatography step. The inactive protein fraction which eluted at low salt consisted primarily of the major cell wall polypeptide plus some

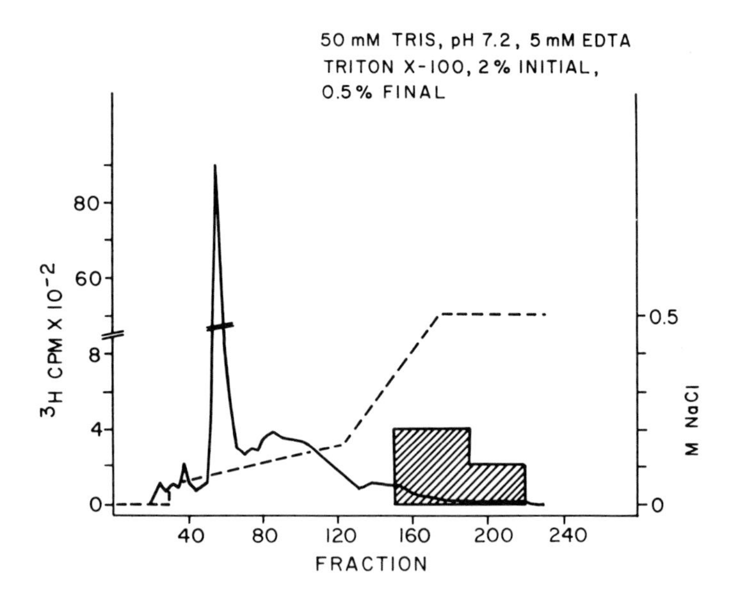

Figure 8 - Chromatography of the Triton-EDTA soluble fraction on DEAE cellulose. The Triton-EDTA soluble fraction (Fig. 7) was precipitated with ethanol, and redissolved in Tris buffer containing Triton X-100 (2 per cent) and EDTA. The sample was applied to a column of Whatman DE52 equilibrated with 2 percent Triton X-100 in the same buffer, and eluted with a NaCl gradient. The Triton concentration was decreased during elution to minimize the amount of Triton in the final receptor fraction and facilitate concentration. Protein is indicated by the solid line, NaCl by the dashed line, and colicin receptor activity by the shaded area.

lower molecular weight material (Fig. 9), and there was no protein which was labeled only with ^3H. The fraction containing the receptor activity also consisted largely of the major cell wall polypeptide peak (Fig. 10), but there was also a protein peak which migrated more slowly than the major peak which appeared to be labeled only with ^3H.

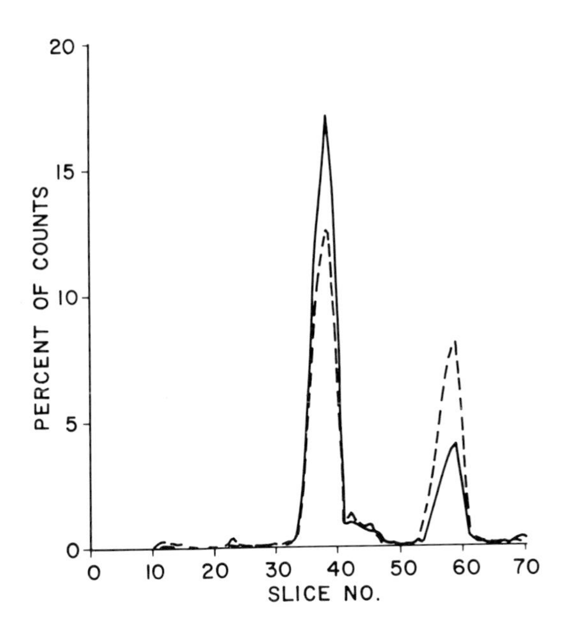

Figure 9 - SDS gel electrophoresis of the inactive protein fraction eluted at low salt from the DEAE column shown in Fig. 8. The solid line represents ^{3}H counts from the sensitive strain and the dashed line represents ^{14}C counts from the resistant strain. Conditions are as in Fig. 6. Reproduced from Reference 11 with permission of the Journal of Biological Chemistry.

At this point an immune precipitation experiment was done to test if this ^{3}H-labeled protein was related to receptor activity. This was done by incubating the receptor fraction from DEAE column I with an excess colicin E_3 and then precipitating the colicin with rabbit antiserum prepared against colicin E_3. This immune precipitate was washed several times, and both the precipitate and the supernatant fractions were examined by SDS polyacrylamide gel electrophoresis. All of the slower-migrating ^{3}H-labeled protein precipitated with the colicin (Fig. 11) while the

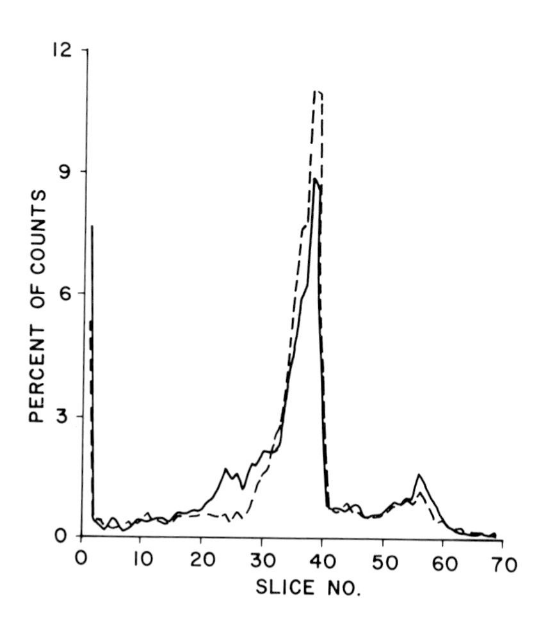

Figure 10 - SDS gel electrophoresis of the receptor fraction eluted at high salt from the DEAE column shown in Fig. 8. The solid line represents ^{3}H counts from the sensitive strain and the dashed line represents ^{14}C counts from the resistant strain. Conditions are as in Fig. 6. Note the small protein peak at about slice 24 that appears to be labeled with ^{3}H but not with ^{14}C. Reproduced from Reference 11 with the permission of the Journal of Biological Chemistry.

supernatant contained only the major cell wall polypeptide peak (Fig. 12). In this experiment about half of the total labeled protein was coprecipitated with the colicin. The gel shown in Fig. 12 is somewhat blurred, probably due to overloading ---- this experiment has now been repeated with more highly purified colicin receptor samples, with the same result (11). Due to the apparent association of the receptor protein with the major cell wall protein

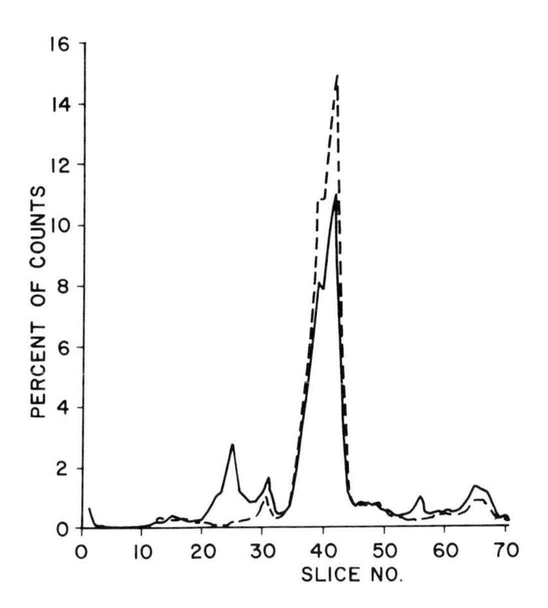

Figure 11 - Immune precipitate of the DEAE column I-purified material shown in Fig. 10. A sample of the receptor fraction was mixed with an excess of colicin E_3, and this was precipitated by the addition of an equivalent amount of rabbit antiserum prepared against purified colicin E_3 (11). The immune precipitate was washed and prepared for SDS gel electrophoresis as in Fig. 6. The solid line represents the ^3H counts from the sensitive strain and the dashed line represents the ^{14}C counts from the resistant strain. About half of the total radioactivity of both isotopes was recovered in the immune precipitate fraction. Note that the ^3H-labeled peak seen in Fig. 10 is roughly doubled in amount and now shows up more clearly.

this procedure offers only at best about a two-fold purification, but it does lend support to the idea that the ^3H-labeled protein seen in Figs. 10 and 11 is involved in a specific way in the colicin receptor

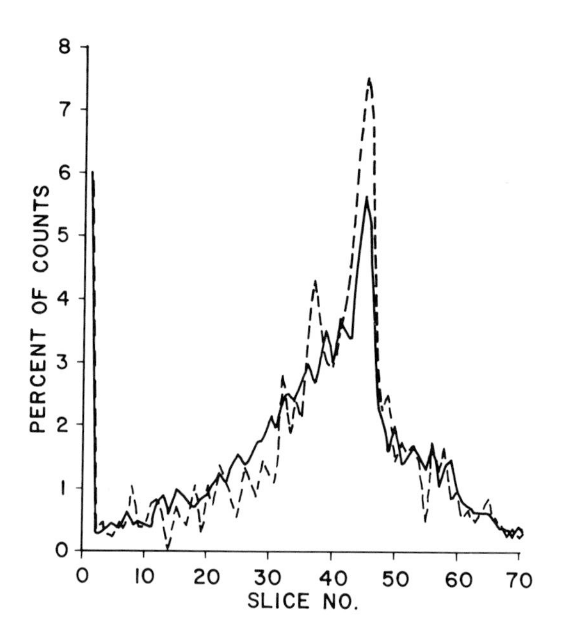

Figure 12 - Immune supernatant from the experiment described in Fig. 11. Note that the ^{3}H-labeled peak appears to be missing from this fraction. The conditions and labeling are as in Figs. 6 and 11.

site.

Further purification of the colicin receptor activity was obtained by precipitating the receptor fraction from DEAE column I with ethanol and redissolving this material in Triton-EDTA solution and applying it to a second DEAE column (DEAE column II). The elution profile of this second column is shown in Fig. 13. A definite peak of radioactive protein eluted with the receptor activity from this column. Fig. 14 shows the profile of the receptor fraction from DEAE column II on a polyacrylamide gel. Again the major protein peak is the major cell wall protein,

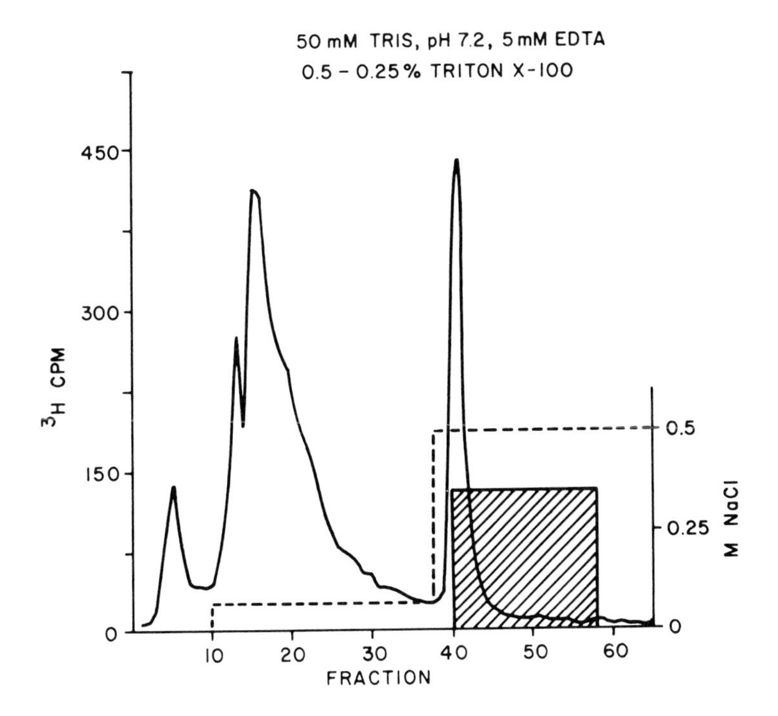

Figure 13 - Chromatography of the receptor fraction from DEAE column I on a second DEAE cellulose column. The receptor fraction from DEAE column I was concentrated by ultrafiltration, precipitated with ethanol, dissolved in Tris buffer containing Triton X-100 and EDTA, and chromatographed essentially as described in the legend of Fig. 8 except that lower Triton concentrations and a stepwise NaCl elution were used. The solid line shows protein, the dashed line shows the NaCl concentration, and the shaded area indicates the fractions containing receptor activity. The fractions containing receptor activity were pooled, concentrated by ultrafiltration, precipitated with ethanol, and redissolved in a small amount of Tris buffer containing Triton X-100.

but now the slower-migrating protein can be seen clearly. This protein is labeled only with ^{3}H, and accounts for 25 percent of the total ^{3}H protein

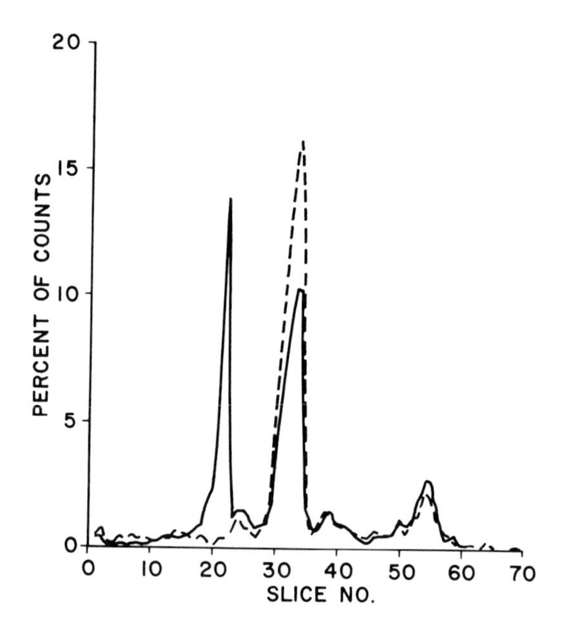

Figure 14 - SDS gel electrophoresis of the receptor fraction eluted from DEAE column II (Fig. 13). The solid line represents ^3H counts from the sensitive culture and the dashed line represents ^{14}C counts from the resistant culture. Conditions are as in Fig. 6. The ^3H-labeled protein seen at slice 21 represents 25 percent of the total ^3H of the gel. Reproduced from Reference 11 with the permission of the Journal of Biological Chemistry.

present on the gel. We have estimated that the molecular weight of this protein is about 60,000 d. as based on a comparison of its mobility on gels to the mobility of known protein standards.

To summarize briefly these results, there are three lines of evidence which indicate that this 60,000 d. protein is a specific component of the colicin E_3 receptor. First, this protein increases from a level which is below detectability on gels to a maximum of about 25 percent as the receptor activity is purified, and during the later stages purification the protein increases in amount roughly in accord with the increase in specific activity of the receptor fraction. Second, in immune precipitation experiments this protein was co-precipitated with colicin by anticolicin. Third, when a resistant culture labeled with ^{14}C amino acids was mixed and cofractionated with a sensitive culture labeled with ^{3}H amino acids this protein was labeled only with ^{3}H, indicating that this protein is missing or altered in the resistant mutant. It should be pointed out that this protein is probably a component of the receptor for all of the group E colicins since the resistant mutant used in this experiment was resistant to colicins E_1, E_2, and E_3.

Role of Carbohydrate in Colicin E_3 Receptor Activity

As noted above, the Triton-EDTA solubilized receptor activity was inactivated by periodate oxidation suggesting that carbohydrate might also be required for receptor activity. This was also found to be true for the purified colicin receptor fraction. Treatment of the purified receptor fraction from DEAE column II with periodate destroyed more than 90 percent of the receptor activity.

In order to see if this periodate sensitivity was due to carbohydrate covalently linked to the 60,000 d. receptor protein we isolated and purified the receptor activity from a culture labeled with ^{3}H amino acids and ^{14}C glucose. The glucose used in this experiment was uniformly labeled, and to minimize "spill" of the glucose label into amino acids the culture was grown with glycerol as a carbon source and as high a level of casamino acids as could be tolerated without a severe reduction in ^{3}H amino acid labeling. This strategy was only partially successful, since there was still considerable "spill" of ^{14}C into protein. In order to correct for this "spill", we isolated protein from the soluble (cytoplasmic) fraction of the broken cells by ammonium sulfate precipitation and applied this to SDS polyacrylamide gels. The ^{14}C and ^{3}H counts in several major peaks observed on these gels were then used to estimate this "spill".

The results of this experiment are shown in Fig. 15 and Table III. When the receptor activity was purified (Table III) there was a progressive enrichment of ^{3}H with respect to ^{14}C. However, the final

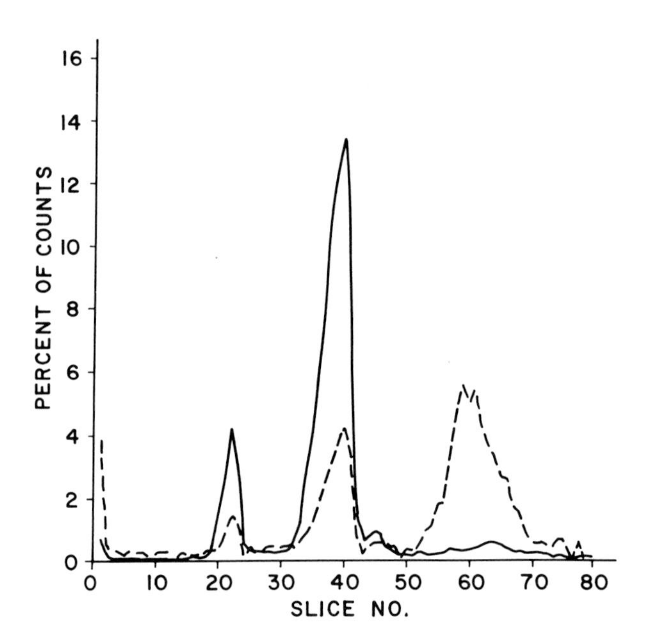

Figure 15 - SDS gel electrophoresis of the receptor fraction purified through the DEAE column II step from a culture labeled with ^{3}H amino acids and ^{14}C glucose. This is the same preparation as shown in Table III. Gel conditions are as in Fig. 6. The solid line represents ^{3}H amino acid label, and the dashed line represents ^{14}C from glucose. Reproduced from Reference 11 with the permission of the Journal of Biological Chemistry.

TABLE III

Purification of E_3 Receptor From Cells Labeled with ^3H-Amino Acids and ^{14}C-Glucose.

Fraction:	Total ^3H Counts	Ratio $^{14}C/^3H$
Crude Envelope	2.8×10^8	0.43
Triton-EDTA Soluble Fract.	7.8×10^7	0.41
DEAE I Fract.	1.3×10^7	0.15
DEAE II Fract.	7.6×10^5	0.12
Receptor band on gel	1.0×10^5	0.043
"Cytoplasmic" protein on gel	--------	0.046

purified fraction from DEAE column 2 still contained more ^{14}C than could be accounted for by "spill" into protein, indicating that there was still some carbohydrate present in the purified fraction. This is also seen in the electrophoretic profile in Fig. 15. There is some ^{14}C in both the receptor protein peak (slice 22) and in the major cell wall polypeptide peak (slice 38), but the amount of ^{14}C with respect to ^3H in these peaks is the same for both peaks and virtually identical to that observed in the cytoplasmic protein. Hence it is unlikely that the receptor protein contains any large amount of covalently bound carbohydrate, although these data are not accurate enough to rule out the presence of a few molecules of sugar bound to the protein. About half of the ^{14}C counts seen on the gel in Fig. 15 were present in a peak which did not contain ^3H-labeled protein (slice 60) and which migrated faster than the major cell wall polypeptide peak. This type of migration is exhibited by unsubstituted lipopolysaccharide "cores" (C. Schnaitman, unpublished), and does suggest that the carbohydrate present in the purified receptor fraction might be lipopolysaccharide. We have also done some preliminary chemical analysis of the carbohydrate found in the purified receptor fraction (11), and these data are also indicative of the presence of lipopolysaccharide or some very similar carbohydrate. However, we have no concrete proof that this carbohydrate is in fact lipopolysaccharide, or that this is the periodate-sensitive component necessary for receptor activity. It is possible that lipopolysaccharide or some similar carbohydrate is necessary in order to maintain the solubilized receptor protein in an active conformation. Lipopolysaccharide does not in itself have receptor activity for colicin E_3 (10).

Other Properties of the Purified Colicin E_3 Receptor

As noted above, the resistant mutant used in identifying the colicin receptor protein (Fig. 14) was resistant to all three group E colicins. Therefore, we were interested to see if the purified receptor fraction still had activity for all three colicins. The results of this experiment are shown in Table IV. The purified preparation is fully active against colicins E_2 and E_3, but has lost almost all activity against colicin E_1. This data suggests that another component (perhaps a second protein or some specific carbohydrate) is also required for the E_1 receptor and that this is lost or inactivated during the purification. This is supported by

TABLE IV

Specificity of Purified E_3 Receptor for Other Colicins

Colicin	Receptor Titer: (Total Units)		
	Triton-EDTA soluble Fraction	Purified receptor (DEAE II fraction)	Percent Recovered
E_1	6.4×10^4	4×10^3	6.3%
E_2	8×10^3	8×10^3	100%
E_3	2.6×10^5	2.6×10^5	100%
K	6.4×10^4	1×10^3	1.6%

genetic evidence (12) that there is a difference between the receptor for colicin E_1 and for colicins E_2 and E_3, although they must share at least one common component. The purified E_3 receptor fraction did not contain receptor activity for colicin K, even though this was present in the Triton-EDTA solubilized starting material (10). This provides further evidence that the receptors for colicin K and the group E colicins are different.

The purified receptor fraction from DEAE column 2 contained all of the receptor activity present in the Triton-EDTA soluble fraction, so it was possible to calculate the number of molecules of the colicin receptor protein per cell. We have calculated that the specific receptor protein identified in Fig. 14 represents 0.044 percent of the total protein of the cell envelope, and based on our measurements of the amount of envelope protein per cell and a molecular weight of 60,000 d. for this protein we have calculated that there are about 220 molecules of this protein per cell. This is based on the assumption that the protein is functional as a monomer of 60,000 d. and must be reduced accordingly if the protein must be present as a dimer, trimer, etc. Although this is a rough estimate, it is interesting that this is close to the number of cytoplasmic membrane-cell wall adhesion sites per cell reported by Bayer (13), and it is tempting to speculate that the colicin E receptor may be located at these adhesion sites. Further studies on the topographic location of the receptors on the cell surface and on the exact mode of penetration and/or action of the group E colicins will be necessary in order to prove this interesting hypothesis.

Acknowledgments

This investigation was supported by Research Grant GB25273 from the National Science Foundation and Research Grant GM18006 and Career Development Award (to CAS) GM22053 from the National Institutes of Health.

Literature Cited

1. Shands, J.W., J. Bacteriol. 90, 266, (1965).
2. Schnaitman, C.A., J. Bacteriol. 108, 553, (1971).
3. White, D.A., W.J. Lennarz, and C.A. Schnaitman, J. Bacteriol. 109, 686, (1972).
4. Schnaitman, C.A., J. Bacteriol. 108, 545, (1971).
5. Levy, S.B., and L. Leive, Proc. Nat. Acad. Sci. U.S.A., 61, 1435, (1968).
6. Braun, V., and K. Rehn, Eur. J. Biochem., 10, 426, (1969).
7. Braun, V., and U. Sieglin, Eur. J. Biochem., 14, 387, (1970).
8. Braun, V., and V. Bosch, Proc. Nat. Acad. Sci. U.S.A., 69, 970, (1972).
9. Bragg, P.D., and C. Hou, Biochim. Biophys. Acta, 274, 478, (1972).
10. Sabet, S.F., and C.A. Schnaitman, J. Bacteriol., 104, 422, (1971).
11. Sabet, S.F., and C.A. Schnaitman, J. Biol. Chem. in press, (1973).
12. Hamon, Y., and Y. Peron, Zentrabl. Bakteriol. Parisitenk. Infektionskr. Hyg. Abt. Orig., 200, 375, (1966).
13. Bayer, M.E., J. Gen. Microbiol. 53, 395, (1968).

MODE OF ACTION OF COLICIN E_3

C.M. Bowman, J. Sidikaro, and M. Nomura

Introduction

Over the past ten years this laboratory has been involved in a continuing study of the action of colicins. More recently, the study has centered on the elucidation of the action of colicin E_3 on a molecular level. The study to be discussed here has attempted to answer the following questions: 1) What is the primary biochemical effect of colicin E_3 on sensitive cells? 2) What defect does E_3 induce in its molecular target? 3) How does the E_3-cell interaction at the receptor site lead to the alteration of the biochemical target? 4) What mechanism has evolved in colicinogenic cells to protect them from the killing action of the colicin they produce? (Cells which produce any kind of colicin are specifically immune to that kind of colicin. This immunity is the primary criterion of colicin classification.) The main strategy of the project has been to identify the biochemical target of this colicin, determine what alteration of the target takes place after E_3 action and then use this information to plan experiments to investigate how E_3 accomplishes its lethal action.

The results of this study show that E_3 specifically inactivates 30S ribosomal subunits. Inactivation results from the cleavage of a small fragment from the three-prime end of the 16S RNA molecule. The identification and characterization of this alteration has allowed the development of a specific chemical assay for E_3 action (that is, the detection of the cleaved fragment). An *in vitro* system has recently been developed in which E_3 causes ribosome inactivation and 16S RNA cleavage. This system holds promise of allowing even more detailed analysis of the action of E_3 in the future. By using this *in vitro* system, it has been possible to show that purified E_3 can induce its specific alteration in the 16S RNA in ribosomes in the absence of non-ribosomal cellular components such as membrane fragments or cytoplasmic enzymes. A study of the relationship between ribosome-inhibiting antibiotics and E_3 action has shown that a group of antibiotics including streptomycin can protect ribosomes from E_3-induced RNA cleavage, both *in vivo* and *in vitro*. The *in vitro* system has allowed investigations into the mechanism of immunity in colicinogenic cells and ultimately in the isolation and purification of the E_3 immunity substance.

Initial Colicin Studies Using Intact Cells

In vivo experiments on whole cells indicate that colicin E_3 affects only protein synthesis (1,2). Treatment of sensitive cells with E_3 (at a multiplicity of 10-50 killing units per cell) leads to a great reduction in the rate of ^{35}S-incorporation into protein, but relatively little change in the synthesis of DNA and RNA, as indicated in Table I (2). E_3 seems to have little or no effect on potassium permeability, respiration, or inorganic phosphate incor-

Table I. Specific Effect of E_3 on Sensitive Cells

Cellular function	Untreated		E_3-treated	
	cpm	%	cpm	%
Incorporation of ^{35}S into protein	1402	100	161	11
Incorporation of ^{14}C into DNA	444	100	562	118
Incorporation of ^{14}C-uracil into RNA	125	100	100	80
^{42}K uptake	4062	100	3612	89
^{42}K leakage	4100	100	5000	122

E. coli strains used were K12W3110 for the protein, DNA and RNA incorporation experiments and B for the potassium transport studies. Experimental data are taken from the original paper (2). Colicin multiplicities were between about 10 and 50 killing units per cell.

poration into several organic phosphate fractions (lipids, acid-soluble nucleotides and acid-insoluble nucleic acids). Thus colicin E_3 is quite different from colicins E_1, E_2, and K which have other, markedly different, effects on sensitive cells (for review, see ref. 3). These results suggest that E_3 primarily and specifically affects the cell's protein synthetic machinery.

Identification of 30S Ribosomal Subunits as the Target of E_3

Konisky and Nomura (4) have shown that ribosomes from E_3-treated cells have very little activity in *in vitro* polypeptide synthesis. In contrast, as shown

Table II. Activity of Protein Synthetic Systems From E_3-Treated and Untreated Cells

Ribosomes	Supernatant	Incorporation (cpm)	%
Control	Control	2160	100
E_3	E_3	177	8
Control	E_3	2318	107
E_3	Control	174	8

Incorporation of ^{14}C-phenylalanine into acid-insoluble protein was assayed in a poly U-directed *in vitro* system. Reaction mixtures contained 1.5 A_{260} units of ribosomes and 1.3 A_{260} units of supernatant fraction as indicated. Reactions proceeded at 37^{0} for 30 min. Data taken from Ref. 4.

in Table II, the supernatant from E_3-treated cells functions normally. Since these inactive ribosomes show normal profiles on sucrose density gradients (4), E_3 must affect a specific target on the ribosome rather than cause generalized ribosome breakdown.

Ribosomes from control (untreated) and E_3-treated cells were dissociated into 50S and 30S subunits, and the protein synthesizing activity was assayed

Table III. Activity of Ribosomal Subunits From E_3-treated and Untreated Cells

50S	30S	Incorporation (cpm)	%
Control	Control	2342	100
E_3	E_3	556	24
Control	E_3	652	28
E_3	Control	2083	89

Ribosomal subunits were prepared from cells which had been treated with E_3 or were untreated. Incorporation of ^{14}C-phenylalanine in a poly U-directed assay system was measured after 30 min. at 37°. Reaction mixtures contained 0.3 A_{260} units 30S and 0.57 A_{260} units 50S subunits. Data taken from Ref. 4.

using the subunits in various combinations as shown in Table 3 (4). The results show that E_3 action leads to the inactivation of 30S ribosomal subunits specifically; this inactivation has little or no effect on the functional capacity of 50S subunits. Although E_3-30S subunits show very little functional activity, their sedimentation pattern on sucrose density gradients is essentially the same as that of control 30S subunits (4). Therefore, E_3 does not cause general ribosomal degradation.

Cleavage of 16S RNA Induced by E_3

Precise identification of the altered molecular component within E_3-30S subunits was initially difficult. However, the 30S ribosomal reconstitution technique developed in our laboratory (6) enabled us to identify the 16S RNA as the only functionally defective component.

The abilities of 16S RNA ("E_3-16S") and total protein fraction ("E_3-TP30") from E_3-treated cells to reconstitute active 30S particles were tested separately as described in Table IV (7). It is clear that E_3-16S forms inactive subunits with either TP30

Table IV. Activity of 30S Ribosomal Subunits Reconstituted from 16S RNA and 30S Ribosomal Proteins (TP30) from Untreated and E_3-treated Cells

16S RNA	TP30	Incorporation (cpm)	%
Control	Control	3812	100
E_3	E_3	195	5
Control	E_3	3920	103
E_3	Control	337	9

Reconstitution mixtures were incubated for 60 min. at 42°. Aliquots were removed and tested for their protein synthetic capacity in a poly U-directed system in the presence of control 50S subunits. Data taken from Ref. 7.

fraction, but that E_3-TP30 as well as control-TP30 is able to produce active 30S subunits when reconstituted with control-16S.

Since the functional defect induced by colicin E_3 in 30S ribosomal subunits resides specifically in the 16S RNA, the RNA was analyzed electrophoretically. It was observed that purified E_3-16S migrates somewhat faster than control-16S RNA on polyacrylamide gels (7). This difference indicates that there is either a size or conformational difference between the two kinds of RNA. To distinguish between these possible explanations, similar gels were run using formaldehyde-denatured RNAs. The mobility difference persisted and both types of RNA migrated much more slowly than the native molecules (Bowman and Nomura, unpublished results). These results suggested that the difference between the molecules was the loss of several nucleotides from the end(s) of the E_3-16S molecule.

To determine the exact nature of this difference, ribonuclease T_1 digests of the two 16S RNAs (^{32}P-labelled) were subjected to two-dimensional electrophoresis "fingerprinting" according to the method of Sanger and co-workers (8,9). Such analysis showed at least four oligonucleotides to be missing from E_3-16S compared to control-16S (7,10). Significantly, the oligonucleotide from the 3'-OH end of the molecule (11) was one of those missing, while the oligonucleotide from the 5'-OH end was present in both RNA.

If the RNA segment were cleaved as one contiguous piece and remained intact during ribosome purification, it might be possible to isolate it directly from ribosomes from E_3-treated cells. Electrophoretic analysis of small molecular weight RNA species from E_3-70S and control-70S showed a discrete new band (designated E_3-fragment) to be present only in the E_3-RNA preparation (7).

The fragment was eluted from the gel, was digested with T_1 ribonuclease-alkaline phosphatase and was fingerprinted. The pattern obtained contained only eight oligonucleotides. Table V shows the compositions of these oligonucleotides (7, and Bowman, Dahlberg and Nomura, unpublished). The small number of

Table V. Comparison of E_3-16S and E_3-fragment Compositions

Oligonucleotide number	Oligonucleotide (after T_1-RNase digestion)	Detected to be absent from E_3-16S	Present in E_3-fragment
10b	AUCAC(UC, UUC, C)A_{OH}	+	+
57b	mUAACAAG	+	+
71	$m_2^6Am_2^6$ACCUG	+	+
69	UAACCG	+	+
54	UUG	–	+
87	UAG	–	+
90	UCG	–	+
108	CG	–	+
	G	–	+

The results are summary of fingerprint analysis of 16S RNA, E_3-16S RNA, and E_3-fragment. The oligonucleotides were assigned numbers by comparison with the fingerprint pattern obtained by Fellner et al. (11). Data are taken from reference 7 and unpublished experiments by C.M. Bowman and J. Dahlberg.

oligonucleotides, all in approximately equimolar amounts, shows that E_3-fragment does not result as a general degradation product from the whole 16S RNA molecule. The presence of spot 10b means that the fragment must originate as the 3'-OH end segment of mature 16S RNA. It is important to note that all of the oligonucleotides which were detected to be missing from E_3-16S are present in E_3-fragment. These results suggest that the cleavage is due to a small number of nucleolytic cleavages (perhaps even one). Santer and Santer recently obtained similar data for the composition of E_3-fragment (12).

Since we have failed to detect any other alteration in E_3-16S RNA, we have concluded that the cleavage of the 16S RNA is the specific effect induced by E_3 and in all likelihood causes the inactivation of the 30S ribosomal subunits. Senior and Holland (13) have recently reported, in contrast to our earlier report (7), that all of the fragment formed by E_3 remains associated with the ribosome rather than dissociating into the supernatant. Our most recent data (though not yet conclusive) still supports the finding that some E_3-fragment dissociates from the ribosomes. Therefore, although we tend to believe that the cleavage itself causes the observed loss in activity, a possibility cannot be excluded that the inactivation of ribosomes is due to dissociation of the fragment rather than the cleavage itself.

Homogeneous E_3-16S RNA and E_3-fragment are useful tools in the study of structure-function relationships of ribosomal RNA. However, the several experiments performed so far in this area are outside the scope of the present discussion.

In Vitro Effect of E_3 on Ribosomes

With the E_3-induced lesion precisely identified, it became possible to try to reproduce the effect of E_3 *in vitro*. Both Boon (14) and our own group (15) reached the same conclusion independently that, under appropriate conditions, purified colicin E_3 will inactivate 70S ribosomes and cleave the 16S RNA.

In our experiments the E_3-fragment produced *in vitro* was isolated and digested with T_1 ribonuclease; the products were fingerprinted. Figure 1 shows a

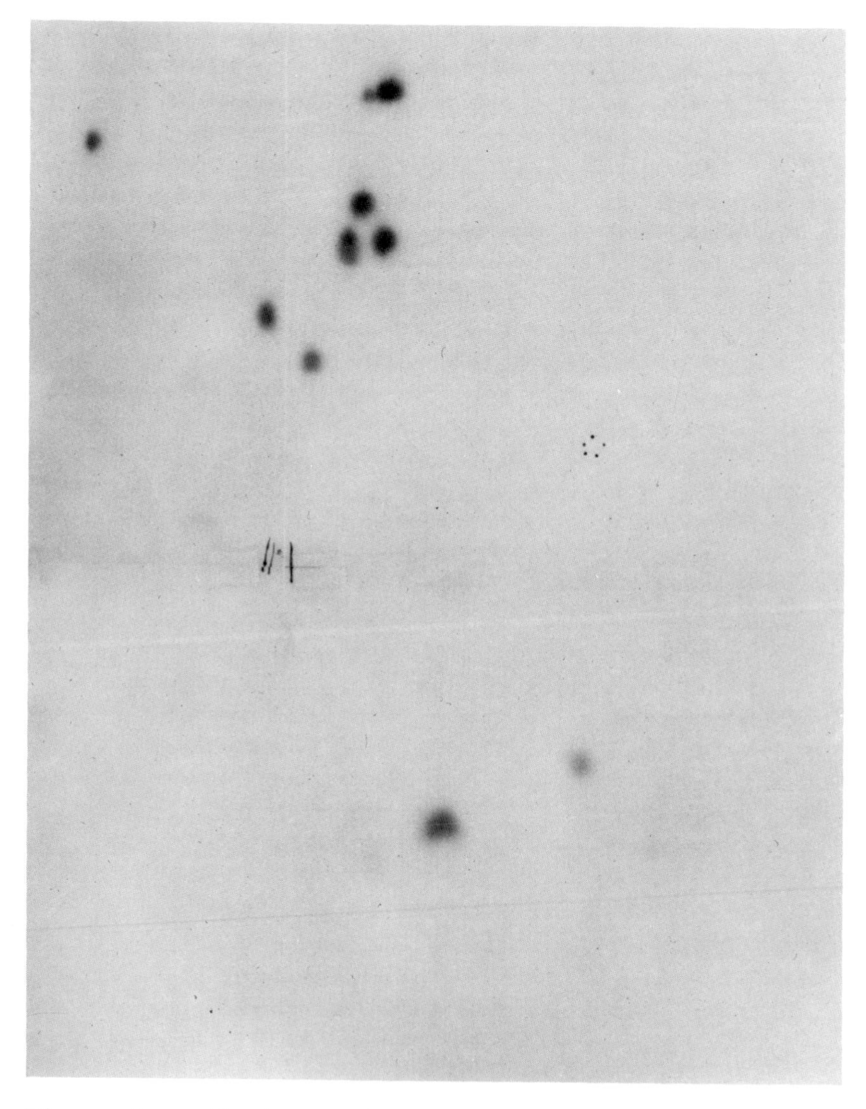

Figure 1a - E_3 fragment was prepared from ribosomes following *in vivo* treatment with E_3. The fragments were purified by electrophoresis on polyacrylamide slab gels. The RNA was digested with T_1 ribonuclease and "fingerprinted" as described in the text. The figures are photographs of the X-ray film autoradiographs.

comparison of the fingerprints of the two types of E_3-fragment; Figure 1a, the in vivo fragment, 1b, the in vitro material. Both fingerprint patterns are the

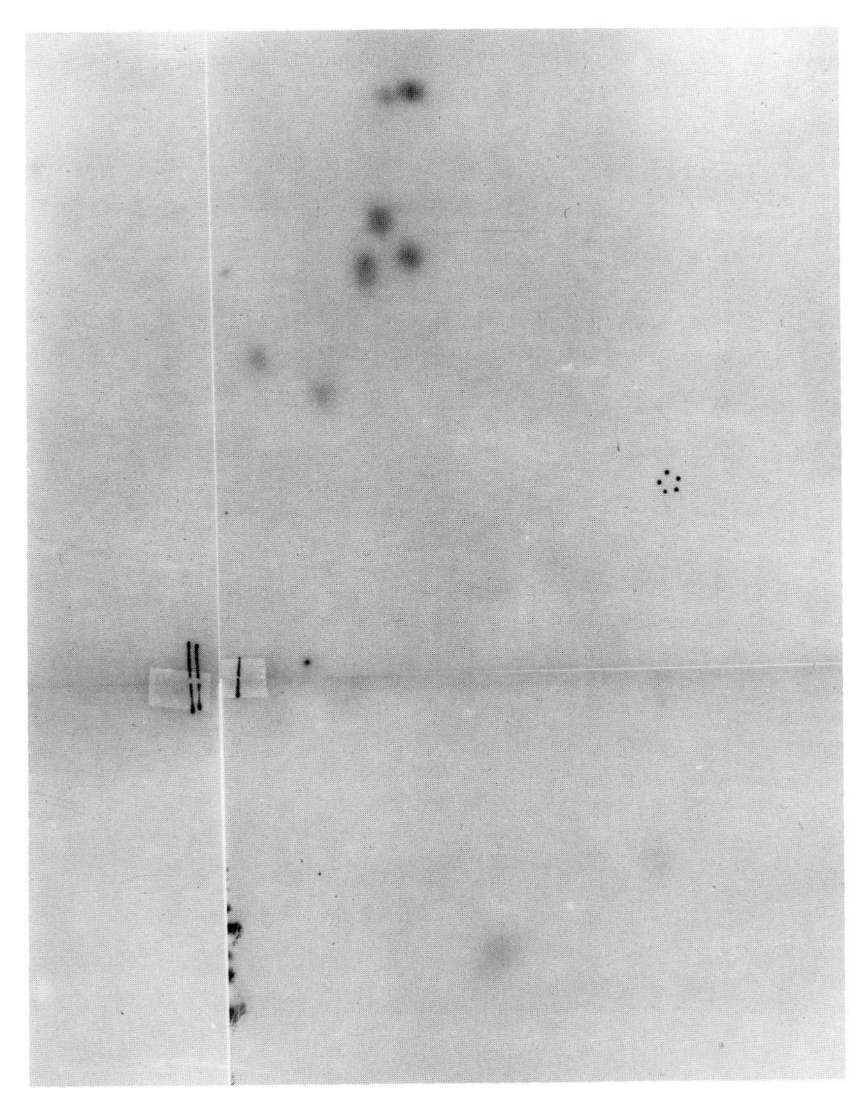

Figure 1b - E_3-fragment was prepared from ribosomes following in vitro treatment with E_3. See Figure 1a for details.

same. Thus, it was concluded that the fragment produced *in vitro* is identical to that produced *in vivo*.

The E_3-induced cleavage of 16S RNA is unique. The site of cleavage on 16S RNA molecules is specific as stated above. Further, T_1 ribonuclease treatment of 30S subunits does not result in the formation of a similar fragment. It was found that E_3 cannot cleave protein-free 16S RNA (15,16); also, E_3 affects 30S ribosomal subunits only in the presence of 50S subunits (16,17). E_3 appears to have no effect on isolated 30S (or 50S) subunits. No known ribonuclease shows such unique "substrate specificity".

Conformation of ribosomes also appears to be important for the cleavage reaction to take place. In collaboration with Dahlberg, Lund, and Kjeldgaard, University of Aarhus, we have examined effects of various known ribosome-antibiotics on the action of E_3 *in vitro* and *in vivo* (18). Streptomycin and several other drugs prevent the E_3-induced cleavage reaction both *in vivo* and *in vitro*. The protection must be specific in nature because streptomycin can only protect cells and ribosomes which are phenotypically streptomycin-sensitive. Streptomycin-resistant cells and their ribosomes (which do not bind the drug) can be affected by E_3, even when streptomycin is present. Thus, streptomycin protection is related to the ribosome's ability to bind the drug. There is no single common mode of action among the antibiotics effective in protection except that all of them interact with 30S subunits. It seems likely that the binding of these antibiotics to 30S subunits may cause some conformational alteration in the 30S subunits, rendering them insensitive to the E_3-induced cleavage reaction. The strong correlation between the patterns of *in vivo* and *in vitro* protection also supports the conclusion that the *in vitro* cleavage reaction is identical to that which takes place *in vivo*.

Isolation of an Inhibitor of E_3 From Immune Cells

The finding that E_3 acts *in vitro* seems to contradict previous experiments (4) which showed that E_3, even at a very high colicin to ribosome ratio, had no effect on ribosomes *in vitro*. However, we have found that the apparent discrepancy is due to the presence of an inhibitor of the *in vitro* cleavage reaction in the crude E_3 preparation which was used in the earlier experiments.

E_3 preparations similar to those used in the first experiments (a crude ammonium sulfate precipitate) were found not to cause the cleavage reaction *in vitro*. Only purified E_3 preparations (purified by passage over a DEAE-Sephadex column (19)) were effective in inducing cleavage of the 16S RNA cleavage. Thus, crude E_3 is not only inactive in cleaving ribosomal RNA, but it also must contain an excess of an inhibitory substance which can prevent the cleavage reaction by added purified E_3.

This inhibitory activity was also found in crude cell extracts from E_3-colicinogenic cells. Such extracts (containing ribosomes) were incubated with purified E_3; no RNA cleavage was observed. However, incubation of ribosomes purified from these extracts (free of cell supernatant) with purified E_3 did result in cleavage (14,15). Furthermore, the ribosome-free cell supernatant ("S-100") from E_3-colicinogenic cells was found to protect purified ribosomes from sensitive cells from E_3-induced cleavage. A similar extract from the non-colicinogenic parent strain showed no such protective activity (15). Thus, it is clear that the presence of the *Col* E_3 factor in a cell confers on it not only the ability to produce E_3, but also the ability to produce a substance which inhibits the action of colicin E_3 on isolated ribosomes *in vitro*. As will be discussed later, this inhibitor could be the immunity substance proposed to explain the mechanism of immunity in colicinogenic cells (1).

Recently the inhibitor has been purified from crude colicin preparations (Sidikaro and Nomura, unpublished results). The crude colicin preparation (ammonium sulfate precipitated) was applied to a column of DEAE-Sephadex and eluted with a gradient of

0 to 0.5 M NaCl. E_3 killing activity was eluted relatively free of the inhibitor at about 0.25 M NaCl. After completion of the gradient, 2 M NaCl was applied to the column. The eluate contained UV-absorbing materials and showed the inhibitor activity.

The fractions showing inhibitor activity were combined and made up to 80% saturation with solid ammonium sulfate. The precipitated material was dissolved and dialyzed against TMAI (10^{-2} M Tris, 10^{-2} M Mg^{++}, 0.03 M NH_4Cl, 6 x 10^{-3} M β-mercaptoethanol). It was then applied to a Sephadex G-50 column which was eluted with TMAI. Figure 2 shows the elution profile of material from this column. Fractions were tested for immunity activity and aliquots of each were electrophoresed on polyacrylamide gels. Only the fractions showing immunity activity showed any bands of material on the gels. This band which did appear was absent in a similar preparation from non-colicinogenic cells. From these observations, material giving this single band is tentatively identified as the inhibitor. This material appears to be primarily protein and very acidic.

Resistance, Tolerance, and Immunity to Colicin E_3

There are three known "biochemical mechanisms" for bacterial cells to be insensitive to colicins. They have been designated resistance, tolerance, and immunity. A cell which fails to adsorb a type of colicin molecule is said to be resistant to it. Most spontaneous mutations in sensitive cells which confer insensitivity involve this type of resistant mutation, presumably due to loss of the specific receptors (see the article by Sabet and Schnaitman in this volume).

Adsorption to a cell receptor is the first step in the killing action of colicins, but it does not necessarily assure the colicin of successful killing. As first observed by Clowes (20) and by ourselves (21), a class of mutants (called tolerant mutants) exists which can adsorb colicins but are still refractory to their effects. Several studies have been

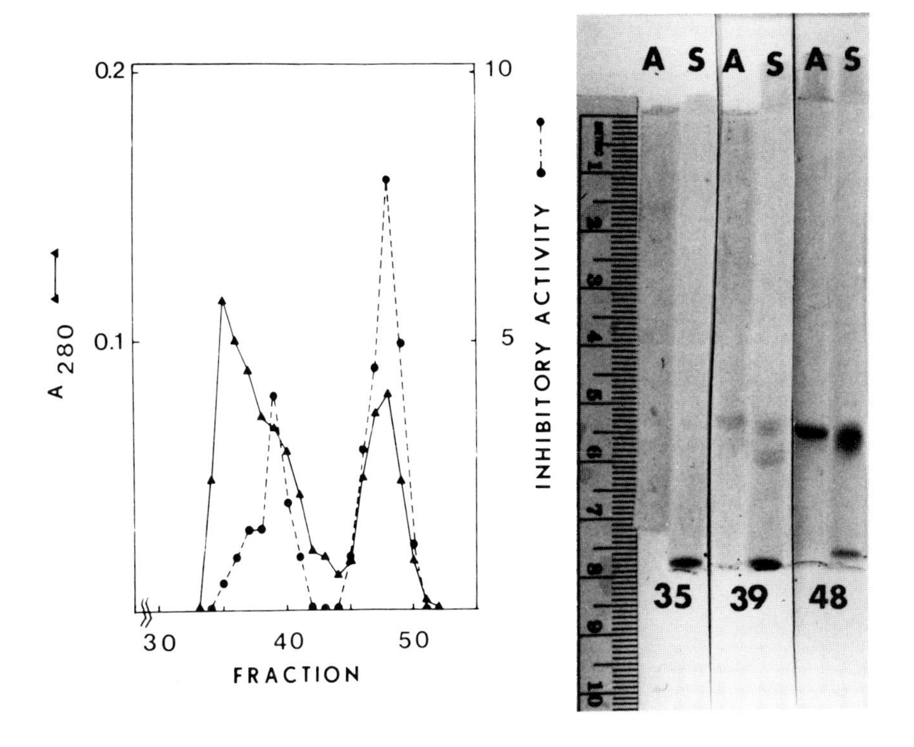

Figure 2 - Purification of the "immunity substance" by Sephadex G-50 chromatography. A column (50 x 1.5 cm) was eluted with TMAI. 0.7 ml fractions were collected. A_{280} of each fraction was measured. "Inhibitory activity" of each fraction was also analyzed as follows: To 1.7 A_{260} 70S and 2.5 μg E_3, 50λ of two fold dilutions of each column fraction was added. The mixtures were incubated at 37° for 60 min, then cooled on ice and assayed for remaining poly U-directed ^{14}C-phenylalanine incorporation activity. One unit of "inhibitory activity" was defined as the amount which gives 50% inhibition of the colicin E_3-induced ribosome inactivation. Fractions were also analyzed by disc gel electrophoresis (0.2 ml aliquots, 10% acrylamide 8 M urea pH 8.7) (34). The gels were sliced longitudinally. One half was stained in 1% Amido black (A) and the other in 0.05% stainsall (S)

(Figure 2, cont'd) (35). The band in the bottom of the three gels is tracking deye. Gel patterns of fraction 35, 39, and 48 are shown as indicated.

made of tolerant mutants (22, 23, 24, 25). It has been suggested that tolerant mutations involve alterations in the cell envelope and that the adsorbed colicin molecule somehow fails to act on the target inside the cell (22, 23).

As has been discussed above, colicinogenic cells are insensitive to the colicin they produce. This insensitivity is called immunity. The exception to this statement, immunity breakdown, occurs only when very large amounts of homologous colicin are added (26, 27, 28).

The particular biochemical target of E_3 is known, its receptor has been isolated and its effect can be reproduced _in vitro_. It is, therefore, a colicin well-suited for study of the mechanism of resistance, tolerance, and immunity. Since resistance appears to be due to the loss of receptors from the cell envelope, ribosomes from resistant mutants should be similar to those of sensitive strains. We treated ribosomes from a resistant mutant strain with E_3 _in vitro_ and found, as expected, that the E_3-fragment was formed, that is, the ribosomes were sensitive to E_3 _in vitro_. We have not tested ribosomes from tolerant mutants as yet. However, we can make definite predictions about the expected results. Most tolerant mutations should affect cell wall or membrane components and have no effect on the ribosomes, leaving them sensitive to E_3; however, there may be a class of mutants with altered ribosome structure which would be insensitive to E_3. Such ribosomal mutants would be extremely valuable in elucidating the normal E_3-ribosome interaction.

As was discussed above, ribosomes from immune cells are sensitive to E_3, but can be protected by the inhibitor we have isolated from immune cells. The inhibitor is produced only in E_3-colicinogenic cells, and is probably responsible for the specific immunity. The inhibitor is present in non-induced colicinogenic cells (15), but its amount in a cell is probably limited. The immunity breakdown mentioned above could be explained by the adsorption of more colicin than can be "neutralized" by the amount of immunity substance present in a colicinogenic cell.

The Mechanism of Action of Colicins

The data discussed above defines the biochemical change produced in sensitive cells by colicin E_3 and strongly indicates that the inactivation of ribosomes by E_3 *in vitro* is very similar to that observed *in vivo*. The 16S RNA cleavage which occurs *in vitro* results from the direct interaction of ribosomes with the colicin molecule in a system apparently free of other cellular components. Thus, the action of E_3 *in vivo* involves, in all likelihood, a direct contact between the E_3 molecule and its target ribosome.

It was previously proposed that colicins in general act from a fixed receptor site located in the cell envelope (2, 21). Two main types of experimental evidence led to this hypothesis. It was found that cells which were treated with colicin K, incubated until an observable biochemical defect appeared, and then were treated with trypsin, could recover from the colicin treatment (29). For example, a cell population which sustained a greater than 95% inhibition of protein synthesis could return to a rate of synthesis of about 50% of the original uninhibited rate within less than two generation time (Bowman and Nomura, unpublished results). This represents an actual rescue of cells in which the effect of the colicin K had clearly taken place. Since trypsin probably does not penetrate into the cytoplasm, the adsorbed, effective colicin K molecules must remain accessible to the trypsin on the "external surface" of the cell. (Of course, the conditions in which trypsin can reverse the inhibition may be limited. It is expected that after longer incubation, for example, secondary damages may become too severe and irreparable.) Since colicin K appears to act directly on the cell surface structure, causing defects in some active transport systems (2, 30, 31), the concept of "action from outside" is still reasonable. However, as discussed before (3), trypsin-reversibility of the inhibition of protein synthesis by E_3 has never been observed; this is consistent with the present conclusion that E_3 acts directly on the ribosomes inside the cell.

A second set of data, involving the location of radioactive colicin in affected cells, also suggested colicin molecules remained at the surface (32). If radioactive colicin E_2 was added to sensitive cells, 90% of the label was ultimately found associated with the membrane and wall fraction of the cell extract. About 60% of the label could be solubilized by trypsin treatment of the cells. Furthermore, only a very small percentage of the radioactive materials were found to be associated with the soluble fraction of the cell. However, as stated in the original article (32), the data do not exclude the possibility of penetration of a single "effective" molecule corresponding to a few per cent of the radioactive E_2 molecules adsorbed by cells (see the article in this volume by Almendinger and Hager, however). It appears, therefore, that there is now no basis to generalize the concept of "action from outside" to all the colicins.

As stated above, colicin E_3 must make specific contact with intracellular ribosomes; it must, therefore, at least partially penetrate the cell envelope. Two possible models for this may be considered: 1) the E_3 molecule penetrates through the cell envelope, but remains associated with it; 2) the E_3 molecule penetrates the cell envelope and is released free into the cytoplasm.

At present, there is little experimental evidence to suggest which model is correct. Since E_3 molecule is large (the molecular weight 60,000), the molecule could probably "reach" from the cell wall into the cytoplasm and the first model is a likely possibility. The model does not need to invoke any special mechanism to release the E_3 molecule from the receptor-E_3 complex. Because it should now be possible to form such receptor-E_3 complexes *in vitro* using the purified E_3-receptor (see the article by Sabet and Schnaitman) and E_3, it would be interesting to see if such receptor-E_3 complexes (which have little killing activity *in vivo*) are able to inactivate ribosomes *in vitro*.

The second model would require that the colicin molecule (or an active portion of it) be freed from its attachment in the cell envelope. This release could include dissociation of the receptor-colicin complex or cleavage of either the receptor or the colicin molecule. Any of these could allow release of the active colicin molecule (or a fragment of it) into the cell cytoplasm. Since diphtheria toxin is cleaved upon entering a cell (33), such a model is not without precedent.

In any case, it seems clear that there are several steps in the RNA cleavage by E_3 *in vivo*, following adsorption of the colicin to the cell receptor. Such treatments as spheroplast formation (which protects cells from killing by both E_3 and E_2 (2)) could prevent the colicin from reaching the cytoplasm. 2, 4-dinitrophenol, also an inhibitor of colicin E_3 which is known to inhibit various membrane-associated transport mechanisms, could probably prevent colicin penetration. Many of the tolerant mutants may involve mutations in the cell membrane or wall which would prevent effective contact of E_3 with ribosomes, without preventing its adsorption to the receptor.

The mechanism just discussed is based only on data for colicin E_3. Although different colicins exert different biochemical effects on sensitive cells, they have nonetheless several common features in their mode of action (1,3). From this point of view, one would now suggest that based on data with E_3, all colicins should interact directly with their targets and modify them chemically. The chemical modification of the targets may or may not be reparable. The evidence presented in this volume by Almendinger and Hager suggests that colicin E_2 probably utilizes endonuclease I as an intermediate in its known biochemical action, that is, the degradation of DNA. However, precise chemical characterization of the primary biochemical event which leads to the E_2-induced DNA degradation has not yet been made. Since E_2 and E_3 are very similar as protein molecules and utilize the same receptor, it would be surprising to see entirely different mechanisms in their primary biochemical actions. Clearly, we must await further studies to solve this problem, and only then could we hope to establish a unified theory on the mode of action of various colicins.

Acknowledgments

We wish to thank our previous co-workers, Dr. A. Maeda and Dr. J. Konisky, who participated in the earlier work on the present colicin E_3 project. Our work was supported in part by the College of Agriculture and Life Sciences, University of Wisconsin, and by grants from the National Institute of General Medical Sciences (BM-15422) and the National Science Foundation (GB-31086X).

References

1. Nomura, M. (1963). Cold Spr. Harb. Symp. Quant. Biol. 28, 315.
2. Nomura, M. and A. Maeda (1965). Zentr. Bakteriol. Parasitenk. Abt. I. Orig. 196, 216.
3. Nomura, M. (1967). Ann. Rev. Microbiol. 21, 257.
4. Konisky, J. and M. Nomura (1967). J. Mol. Biol. 26, 181.
5. Konisky, J. (1968). Ph.D. Thesis, University of Wisconsin.
6. Traub, P. and M. Nomura (1968). Proc. Nat. Acad. Sci. U.S. 59, 777.
7. Bowman, C.M., J.E. Dahlberg, T. Ikemura, J. Konisky, and M. Nomura (1971). Proc. Nat. Acad.

Sci. U.S. 68, 964.
8. Sanger, F., G.G. Brownlee, and B.G. Barrell (1965). J. Mol. Biol. 13, 373.
9. Brownlee, G.G. and F. Sanger (1967). J. Mol. Biol. 23, 337.
10. Senior, B.W. and I.B. Holland (1971). Proc. Nat. Acad. Sci. U.S. 68, 959.
11. Fellner, P., C. Ehresman, and J.P. Ebel (1970). Nature 225, 26.
12. Santer, U.V. and M. Santer (1972). FEBS Letters 21, 311.
13. Senior, B.W. and I.B. Holland (1972). Journ. Supramolec. Struc. 1, 135.
14. Boon, T. (1971). Proc. Nat. Acad. Sci. U.S. 68, 2421.
15. Bowman, C.M., J. Sidikaro, and M. Nomura (1971). Nature New Biology 234, 133.
16. Boon, T. (1972). Proc. Nat. Acad. Sci. U.S. 69, 549.
17. Bowman, C.M. (1972). FEBS Letters 22, 73.
18. Dahlberg, A.E., E. Lund, N.O. Kjeldjaard, C.M. Bowman, and M. Nomura, manuscript submitted for publication.
19. Herschman, H.R. and D.R. Helinski (1967). J. Biol. Chem. 242, 5360.
20. Clowes, R.C. (965). Zentr. Bakteriol. Parasitenk. Abt. I. Orig. 196, 152.
21. Nomura, M. (1964). Proc. Nat. Acad. Sci. U.S. 52, 1514.
22. Nagel de Zwaig, R. and S. Luria (1967). J. Bact. 94, 1112.
23. Nomura, M. and C. Witten (1967). J. Bact. 94, 1093.
24. Reeves, P. (1966). Australian J. Exptl. Biol. Med. Sci. 44, 301.
25. Hill, C. and I.B. Holland (1967). J. Bact. 94, 677.
26. Fredericq, P. (1957). Ann. Rev. Microbiol. 11, 7.
27. Fredericq, P. (1958). Symp. Soc. Exptl. Biol. 12, 104.

28. Levisohn, R., J. Konisky, and M. Nomura (1968). J. Bact. 96, 811.
29. Nomura, M. and M. Nakamura (1962). Biochem. Biophys. Res. Comm. 7, 306.
30. Luria, S.E. (1964). Ann. Inst. Pasteur 107, supplement to No. 5, 67.
31. Fields, K.L. and S.E. Luria (1969). J. Bact. 97, 57.
32. Maeda, A. and M. Nomura (1966). J. Bact. 91, 685.
33. Uchida, T., D.M. Gill, and A.M. Pappenheimer, Jr. (1971). Nature New Biology 233, 8.
34. Davis, B.J. (1964). Ann. N.Y. Acad. Sci. 121, 404.
35. Dahlberg, A.E., C.W. Dingman, and A.C. Peacock. (1969). J. Mol. Biol. 41, 139.

STUDIES ON THE MECHANISM OF ACTION OF COLICIN E_2

Rosemary Almendinger and Lowell P. Hager

Colicin E_2 is probably the best studied colicin insofar as total volume of research is concerned. However, until recently, it's mechanism of action was no better understood than that of any other colicin. Most of the published work on E_2 has been concerned with observations on the events occurring in normal sensitive cells after colicin adsorption (1). Techniques for modifying the cell surface have recently been developed and these have now been used to help elucidate the mechanism for colicin action (2). In this paper, we report new work on reconstitution experiments involving the interaction of colicin E_2 and endonuclease I with spheroplast preparations.

GENERAL CONSIDERATIONS

Much of the interest in colicin E_2 stemmed from early studies in Nomura's laboratory which indicated that the colicin remained exterior to the cell membrane while causing internal damage and cell death (3). This conclusion came both from the fact that E_2-treated cells could be rescued from death by trypsin treatment (3-5), and from binding studies with radioactive colicin which showed that only one percent of the colicin could be found in the cell super-

Abbreviations: DNA, deoxyribonucleic acid; RNA, ribonucleic acid; DNP, 2,4-dinitrophenol; DNase, deoxyribonuclease; tRNA, transfer RNA; RNase, ribonuclease; Tris, tris (hydroxymethyl) aminomethane; EDTA, ethylene diaminetetra acetic acid; KU, killing units; dAT, poly-deoxyadenylic-thymidylic acid; ATP, adenosine triphosphate.

natant fraction whereas the remainder was mostly in the cell envelope fraction (3).

Nomura's work showed that DNA and RNA synthesis is inhibited shortly after adsorption of colicin E_2 and also that protein synthesis ultimately is stopped (4). However, the extrachromosomal machinery in cells treated with low levels of E_2 appears intact since T_4 and T_5 phage can multiply in such cells and lysogenic λ also can produce near normal bursts after E_2 induction (4). At the same time, Nomura showed that the primary biochemical lesion resulting from E_2 binding to sensitive cells was both an inhibition of DNA synthesis and a degradation of chromosomal DNA to acid soluble products (4,6,7). His results showed that the addition of E_2 to sensitive cells caused DNA degradation after a 5 to 30 minute lag. The extent of the lag period and also the rate of degradation was dependent on E_2 multiplicity. However, the addition of one killing unit per cell was sufficient to induce extensive degradation of DNA to acid soluble products. This work has since been confirmed in many other laboratories (8-10).

DNA degradation in E_2-treated cells can be inhibited by the addition of dinitrophenol, cyanide, 8-hydroxyquinoline or by the addition of colicin K simultaneous with the colicin E_2 (4,6,8,11-14). Trypsin treatment can restore cell viability at any time up to at least 2 hours after the simultaneous addition of DNP and E_2 to sensitive cells (5,12). However, simultaneous addition of E_2 and chloramphenicol or streptomycin to sensitive cells cannot inhibit the killing effect of E_2. Starvation of the cells for amino acids also does not prevent E_2 induced killing (4,8). These results are interpreted to indicate that no new DNase or other protein is being synthesized after colicin adsorption. Recent evidence by Holland indicates that DNA synthesis also is not necessary for the development of the lethal effects of E_2. Holland has shown that neither the addition of nalidixic acid to sensitive cells nor thymine starvation in a thymine requiring strain have an inhibitory effect on E_2 induced DNA degradation (6,8). In short, energy metabolism seems to be the only metabolic requirement for supporting the lethal actions of colicin E_2.

Approximately one year ago, Ringrose and Mizuno independently published data on the mode of DNA degradation in cells treated with high multiplicities of colicin E_2 (9,10). Their data are summarized in Table I. Several differences can be noted in the two

TABLE I

Mode of DNA Degradation

Type of Cleavage	Cells + E_2		Endonuclease I	
	Ringrose	Mizuno	Pure	tRNA Inhibited
Single strand endonuclease	+	-	-	+
Double strand endonuclease	+	+	+	±
Exonuclease	+	+	+	-

reports. However, there is general agreement that the sequence of events leading to acid soluble products begins with the appearance of many double strand cleavages in the DNA. Shortly after the initiation of double strand cleavages, a rapid exonuclease activity occurs. The first double strand cleavage would be a lethal event for the cell since no repair mechanism is known for double strand breaks in DNA. It is interesting to note in the case of E_2 that the first double strand cleavages in DNA appear simultaneously with the loss of trypsin reversibility (9,10). In E_2 induced DNA degradation, double strand nicks continue to appear until the DNA has reached a limit molecular weight of about 2×10^6 daltons; then the exonuclease activity rapidly takes over. During the exonuclease phase, no DNA species in the molecular weight range between 5,000 and 1×10^6 daltons can be found in the cells. The time of initiation for each degradative event in this series depends on the multiplicity of the colicin. However, the sequence of events is identical at all multiplicity levels of E_2.

Mizuno and others have also reported that extensive ribosomal RNA degradation occurs in E_2 treated cells (9,14-17). However, RNA degradation requires that the cells be grown on a specific medium and RNA degradation in response to E_2 is not a general phenomenon. An interesting outcome from this work is that whereas trypsin treatment cannot stop DNA degradation in cells which have been incubated with E_2 for more than 5 minutes, trypsin treatment can prevent RNA degradation in the same cells provided that the trypsin is added within a 15 minute period after colicin addition (14). Trypsin reversibility of the RNA degradation is lost, though, by 30 minutes when the RNA degradative products begin to appear. This observation lends support to Nomura's original hypothesis that the E_2 colicin remains on the cell exterior while causing some type of message to be sent inside the cell (6,7). In the case of the cells which degrade both DNA and RNA in response to E_2, two messages appear to be sent; an early one for DNA degradation and a later one for RNA degradation. However, in either case, once the message is sent, the resulting biochemical lesion would be trypsin irreversible.

Two years ago our laboratory started work on the hypothesis that endonuclease I is the intermediary message which colicin E_2 uses to initiate chromosomal DNA degradation. Endonuclease I is an enzyme which occurs in the periplasmic space of the cell (18-21). Periplasmic space may be an actual storage area for degradative enzymes and may lie between the membrane and cell wall as is pictured in Figure 1, or it may be only a mechanistic definition for a collection of proteins which are loosely associated with the cytoplasmic membrane and which therefore can be easily released from the membrane into the external environment (22-26).

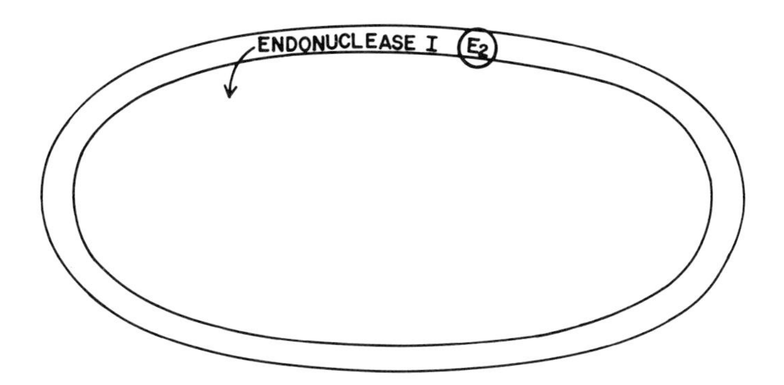

Figure 1 - Mode of action of colicin E_2.

Endonuclease I can bind with and be inhibited by both ribosomal and tRNA (27-29). Endonuclease I appears to exist in the periplasmic space in such an inhibited form (20,21), complexed with tRNA. Table I summarizes the DNase activities associated with this enzyme. Pure endonuclease I produces double strand cleavages in native DNA (27,29-32), and Lehman has also shown it to have a sizable exonuclease activity (30). When inhibited by being complexed with tRNA, endonuclease I does not degrade DNA extensively by any of these mechanisms. However, Helinski (33) has shown that under high salt conditions, the tRNA inhibited enzyme is capable of producing a few single strand breaks in DNA. Thus, endonuclease I could cause any or all of the DNA breakages seen in cells after colicin E_2 challenge.

There is some evidence in earlier literature which indicates that endonuclease I could be involved in E_2 directed DNA degradation. Two different treatments of cells which affect periplasmic endonuclease have been shown to decrease the E_2 sensitivity of cells. Nomura found that spheroplasts are totally insensitive to E_2 and he also showed that spheroplast DNA is not degraded after E_2 binding (6). Spheroplast formation under the conditions used by Nomura should release 95-100% of the endonuclease I from the cell (20, and our unpublished results). Further,

Beppu and Arima (34) showed that cells which have been plasmolyzed with salt or sucrose also are more resistant to E_2 induced killing and DNA degradation. The plasmolysis vacuole of *E. coli* tends to occur in the polar regions of the cell (35) and it is this area which contains the major portion of the periplasmic enzymes (25,36). Upon plasmolysis, the vacuole appears and the components of the incubation medium can flood the area. The incubation medium used both by Nomura and by Beppu and Arima in their studies was Penassay Broth. We have found that Penassay Broth contains a potent inhibitor for endonuclease I and this may interfere with the normal E_2 killing process. The endonuclease I inhibitor in Penassay medium is not removed by incubation with 500 μg ribonuclease per ml for 30 minutes at 37°C. A second hint of evidence for the involvement of endonuclease I in E_2 induced DNA degradation comes from the work of Mizuno. Mizuno found that cells which are incubated with colicin have normal endonuclease levels. However, he also found that endonuclease from E_2 treated cells needs much less RNase treatment to strip it of inhibitory RNA and thus activate it for DNA hydrolysis (9). Mizuno explained this result as being due to E_2 induced RNA degradation in the cells. However, tRNA is little affected by E_2 treatment (15,16) although it is the most potent RNA inhibitor of endonuclease (28). Instead, Mizuno's findings implied to us that at least some of the inhibitory tRNA had been removed in the treatment of cells with E_2 and replaced by DNA. In this case, the endonuclease would be quite active on DNA substrates in the absence of RNase treatment. This argument in turn led to the hypothesis that endonuclease I might be part of or all of the E_2 message.

Experiments with Endonuclease Deficient Cells

Our initial approach to studying the possible implication of endonuclease I in the colicin E_2 mechanism was to employ the osmotic shock procedure developed in Heppel's laboratory. Periplasmic enzymes are released from cells by osmotic shock, thus leading to the preparation of endonuclease deficient cells (19,21). Differing amounts of various periplasmic enzymes can be released depending on the conditions used in the shock. The Heppel shock procedure is carried out in two stages: the first stage consists of an incubation of the cells in Tris-EDTA buffer with varying levels of sucrose; the second stage consists of a quick resuspension of first stage cells in cold water containing varying amounts of $MgCl_2$. With high sucrose concentrations in Stage 1 and high concentrations of $MgCl_2$ in Stage 2, maximal amounts of endonuclease I are released from the cell. Several periplasmic phosphatases, including a hexose acid phosphatase, are released in quite low levels using these conditions. When lower concentrations of both sucrose and $MgCl_2$ are used in the two stage osmotic shock, the release of endonuclease I is minimal and the release of the phosphatases are maximal. Table II shows the levels of two periplasmic enzymes which are released when different shock conditions are used. Inorganic pyrophosphatase, a cytoplasmic enzyme, which is not released by osmotic shock was measured (38) and served as a monitor to detect cell lysis. During osmotic shock, the cells remain viable (2,37,38) and little lysis occurs. The levels of the

TABLE II

Osmotic Shock Conditions			Enzyme Release		
	% Sucrose in Stage I	$MgCl_2$ Conc. in Stage II	Endonuclease I	Acid Phosphatase	Inorganic Pyrophosphatase
			Units/10^{10} Cells	Units/10^{10} Cells	Units/10^{10} Cells
1.	0	5×10^{-4} M	0	700	0
2.	5	5×10^{-4} M	235	2430	8
3.	20	5×10^{-4} M	1036	1650	72
4.	20	2×10^{-2} M	1418	740	81
5.	Sonic oscillated control		1435	2180	1,320

various enzymes released by differential shock can be compared with the total level of the enzyme in the cell as shown on the bottom line of Table II. The osmotic shock procedure not only releases periplasmic proteins from the cell, it also releases acid-soluble nucleotide pools and one half of the total cell wall lipopolysaccharide (39-43). Since both of these components are also lost when no sucrose is present in the first stage of the osmotic shock, treatment of cells in the absence of sucrose served as a control to determine if either of these latter components might affect colicin action. Periplasmic enzyme release is neglible when sucrose is omitted from the osmotic shock (Table II).

When E_2 sensitive cells were subjected to each of these osmotic shock treatments and then tested for sensitivity to colicin E_2, it was found that under certain conditions there was an increased resistance to E_2 killing. The increased resistance was proportional to the amount of endonuclease I released and did not correlate with the release of any other material. Figure 2 shows the data upon which this conclusion is based. Curve D is the survival curve for normal untreated sensitive cells. Curve E represents the survival curve for cells treated only with Tris-EDTA. There is no difference between curves D and E. Thus, the release of lipopolysaccharide and the loss of the nucleotide pools from the cell have no effect on E_2 killing. However, when perceptable levels of endonuclease I are released by osmotic shock, the survival curves reflect the increased resistance of these cells to E_2 killing. When 97 per cent of the endonuclease I is released (Curve A), maximal resistance to E_2 is obtained. In contrast, when 100 per cent of the hexose acid phosphatase is released along with minimal levels of endonuclease I, (Curve C), the survival curve is almost identical to that of the controls.

The rate of DNA degradation after E_2 adsorption to osmotic shocked cells is also affected by the release of endonuclease I during the osmotic shock as seen in Figure 3. Curve C in Figure 3 shows the amount of DNA degradation which occurs in normal cells

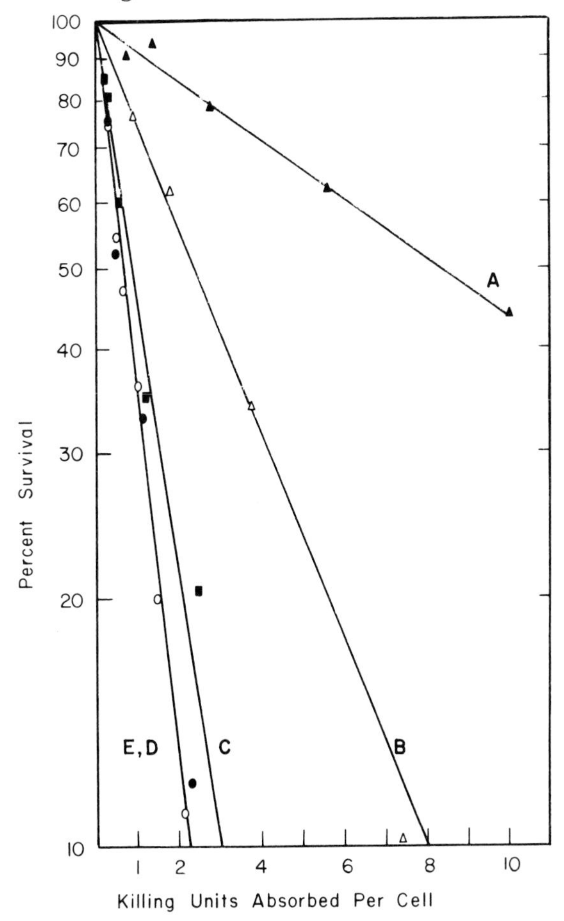

Figure 2 - Sensitivity of osmotical shocked cells to colicin E_2. Untreated cells = Curve D (o—o). EDTA-treated cells = Curve E (●—●). Shocked cells with 5% sucrose-EDTA followed by 5 x 10^{-4}M $MgCl_2$ = Curve C (■—■). Shocked cells with 20% sucrose-EDTA followed by 5 x 10^{-4}M $MgCl_2$ = Curve B (△—△). Shocked cells with 20% sucrose-EDTA followed by 2 x 10^{-2}M $MgCl_2$ = Curve A (△—△). See reference for details.

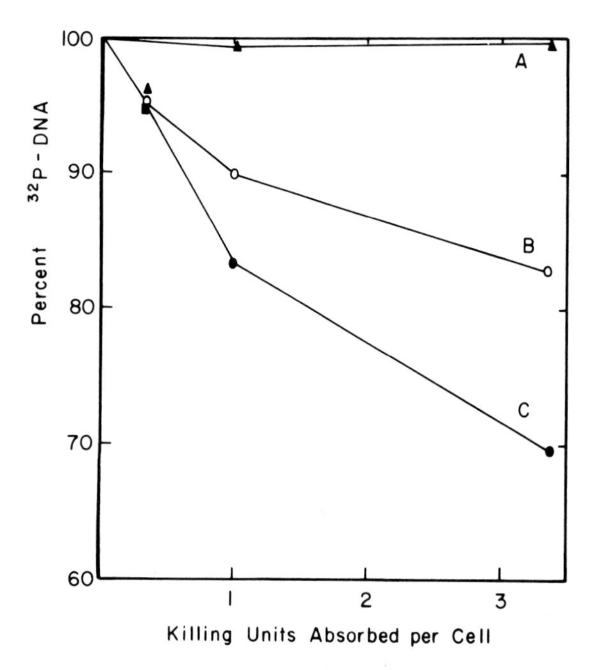

Figure 3 - Acid insoluble DNA remaining after a 50 minute colicin E_2 treatment of osmotic shocked cells. Normal cells = Curve C (●—●). EDTA-treated cells = Curve B (o—o). Shocked cells with 20% sucrose-EDTA followed by 2 x 10^{-2}M $MgCl_2$ = Curve A (▲—▲). See reference for details.

during a 50 minute incubation with varying levels of colicin. Curve B shows the E_2 induced DNA degradation in cells pre-treated with Tris-EDTA alone. Under these conditions, all of the endonuclease I remains with the cell. Curve A reflects the DNA content of cells which have lost 97 per cent of their endonuclease I by osmotic shock before colicin E_2 adsorption. It is readily apparent that no detectable degradation has occurred in these endonuclease deficient cells.

We looked for other possible explanations for the resistance to E_2 in osmotic shocked cells but could find none. Oxidative phosphorylation in shocked cells appears intact and binding of the colicin occurs at normal levels (unpublished results).

Our next line of investigation was to look at colicin sensitivity of E. coli strains which were made endonuclease deficient through mutation (44). Mizuno (9) had previously shown that the type and rate of DNA degradation occurring in strain 1100, an endonuclease I deficient strain, was the same as it's parent, strain 1000, in the presence of 100 E_2 killing units per cell. However, when we looked at cell survival of these two strains at low multiplicity levels of colicin E_2, we could see a dramatic difference between the mutant and the parent strain. Figure 4A compares the E_2 susceptibility of early log phase cells for the mutant (Curve 1), it's parent (Curve 2), and W3110 Sm^r (Curve 3), our normal assay strain. The mutant cells, in early log phase, are not only more resistant to E_2 when compared to the parent cells, but also show a multiple hit killing curve. With older cells, the differences between parent and mutant cells gradually disappear. After 2 generations into late log phase, the mutant cells show the same survival curve as the parent cells. In comparison, colicin I_b, an oxidative phosphorylation inhibitor (45) produces the same identical killing curve with early log cells of both strains (Figure 4B). The parent strain is considerably more resistant to both colicin E_2 and I_b when compared to our normal assay strain, W3110. No apparent reason could be found for this difference in sensitivity. Neither the parent nor the mutant harbored col factor plasmids since neither strain could be induced to produce a colicin, and all 3 strains, mutant, parent and assay strain, adsorbed similar amounts of both colicins.

Table III shows the endonuclease I levels of the normal assay strain (W3110 Sm^r), the endonuclease deficient strain 1100, and the parent strain 1000 at various stages of growth. Endonuclease I activity was measured with two different substrates, ^{32}P labeled E. coli DNA and ^3H-labeled poly dAT (21). It was found that the levels of endonuclease I in the mutant are dependent upon the substrate used in the

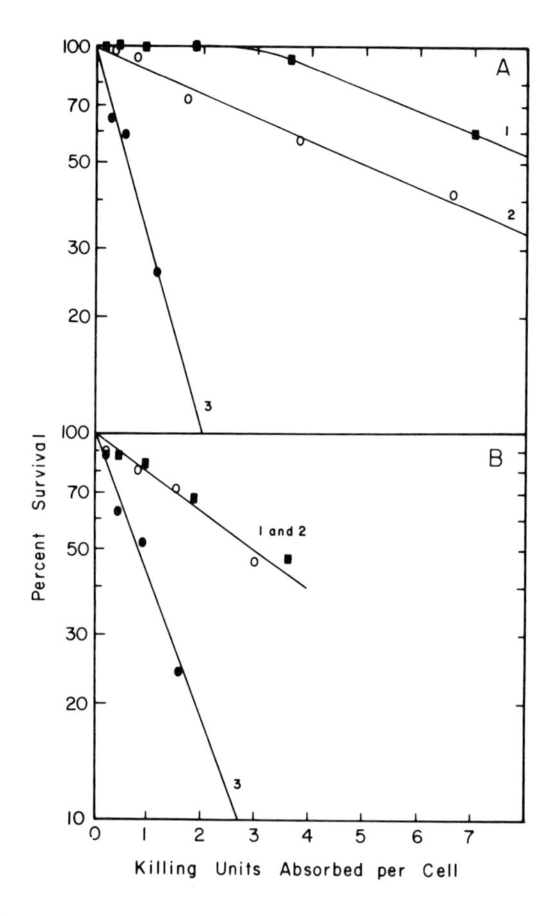

Figure 4 - Colicin sensitivity of an endonuclease I deficient strain. Figure A is for colicin E_2 and Figure B for colicin I_b. The endonuclease I minus mutant (1100) is represented by curves labeled 1 (■—■); it's parent (1000) by curves labeled 2 (o—o) and the normal assay strain W3110 Sm^r by curves labeled 3 (●—●). See reference for details.

assay. The endonuclease I level of the mutant is only 1 per cent of the parent level when E. coli DNA is used but is 20 per cent when poly dAT is used as substrate. The endonuclease levels of the mutant strain not only vary with the substrate used in the

TABLE III

Endonuclease I Content of Several Strains of *Escherichia coli* at Three Stages of Growth

E. coli strain	Growth phase	Cell Density at time of harvest	Endonuclease I Activity		
			^{32}P-labeled DNA	^{3}H-labeled poly d AT	Ratio $\frac{\text{poly d AT}}{\text{DNA}}$
		Cells/ml	Units/10^{10} Cells	Units/10^{10} Cells	
1. W 3110 Sm^r	very early log	2×10^8	20.8	257	12
2. "	early log	5×10^8	20.7	204	10
3. "	mid log	9×10^8	6.3	187	3
4. 1000	very early log	2×10^8	37.4	620	17
5. "	early log	5×10^8	16.7	500	30
6. "	mid log	9×10^8	12.8	258	20
7. 1100	very early log	2×10^8	0.38	120	316
8. "	early log	5×10^8	0.90	172	191
9. "	mid log	9×10^8	0.69	202	293

assay and the age of the cells (Table III), but also with the composition of the growth medium (unpublished results). In fact, when the mutant is grown in a rich medium, it shows a negative endonuclease activity. That is, the mutant extract has higher DNase activity when inhibited with tRNA than when activated with ribonuclease. Thus, it appears that the endonuclease "deficient" mutant is really a mutant which possesses an endonuclease having altered characteristics. The altered endonuclease may be present in the mutant in some growth phases at much higher levels than was previously thought. Current work in our

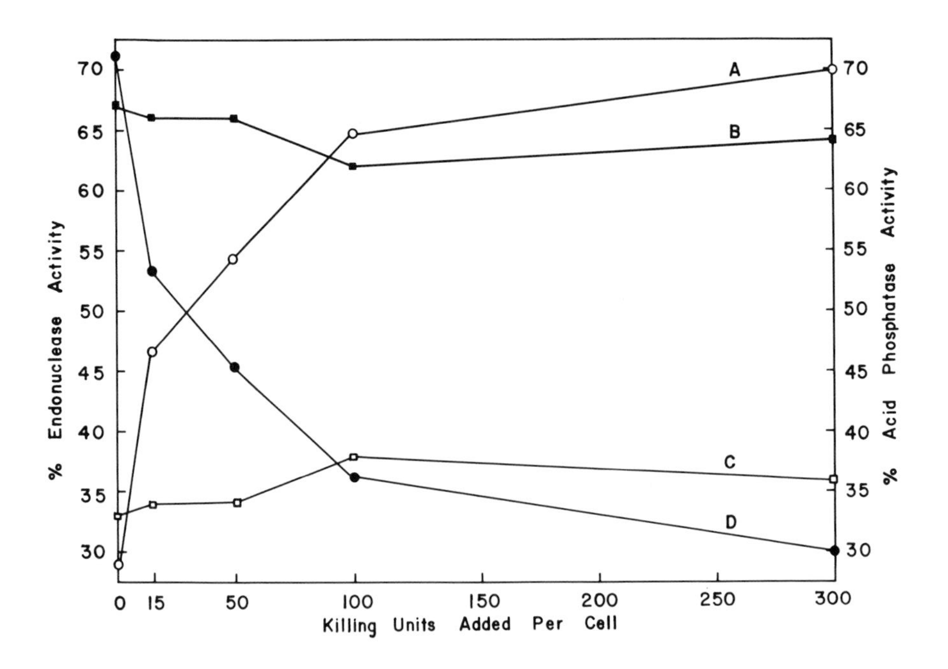

Figure 5 - Release of periplasmic enzymes by spheroplast formation after colicin E_2 adsorption. Endonuclease I released = Curve D (●—●). Endonuclease I retained by cells = Curve A (○—○). Acid phosphatase released = Curve B (■—■). Acid phosphatase retained by cells = Curve C (□—□). See reference 2 for details.

laboratory, is aimed at clarifying this situation. However, even if only 5 per cent of the total endonuclease content of the parent strain is present in the mutant, this 5 per cent level would be sufficient to kill the cell and induce extensive DNA degradation. The evidence which supports this conclusion will be discussed later.

As indicated above, endonuclease I can be released from the cell during the process of spheroplast formation using EDTA-lysozyme treatment (18-20). Figure 5 shows, however, that cells which have previously been incubated with colicin E_2 release less endonuclease I than do untreated cells when both are converted to spheroplasts under identical conditions. Curve D shows the levels of endonuclease I released from cells treated with increasing levels of colicin before spheroplast formation. At E_2 multiplicities between 0 and 100, the degree of release is inversely proportional to the amount of colicin added. Cells treated with E_2 show correspondingly higher amounts of endonuclease I remaining with the cells (Curve A). The endonuclease remaining with the cells can be detected in the soluble fraction either after osmotic lysis or a 90 second treatment in a sonic oscillator. Acid phosphatase, another periplasmic enzyme, does not show this difference in behavior between untreated and colicin E_2-treated cells. Acid phosphatase is released in identical amounts, independent of E_2 treatment, as is shown by Curve B. Curve C shows the amount of acid phosphatase which remains associated with the cell. These results therefore indicate that the endonuclease I response to E_2 is not just due to a general inhibition of periplasmic enzyme release. Rather, this effect appears specific just for periplasmic endonuclease I. The degree of retention of endonuclease I by colicin-treated cells is dependent not only on colicin concentration but also on other factors. For example, the type of EDTA used in the lysozyme treatment is important. As a result, we do not consistently see the same extent of response to the colicin as shown in Figure 5. However, there is always at least a 10-20 per cent decrease in the amount of endonuclease I released from E_2 treated cells as measured by conversion of the cells to spheroplasts.

Reconstitution Experiments

At this point in our investigation, the colicin E_3 experiments of Boone and Bowman and Nomura (46-49) were published. These results indicate that E_3 can act directly on the ribosomes. Both groups showed that the incubation of E_3 and ribosomes could produce in vitro the same specific cleavage induced in the 16S RNA of the 30S ribosome by E_3 under in vivo conditions. Several investigators had previously indicated that E_2 can not catalyze in vitro DNA degradation (4,10,50,51) but we felt we also had to reinvestigate this possibility. We have attempted to measure DNA degradation in the presence of highly purified E_2 both by the appearance of acid soluble products and by shifts in the DNA peak on alkaline sucrose gradients. We have used as substrates in these studies, pure E. coli DNA, poly dAT and also E. coli DNA bound in situ to cell membranes. This latter DNA was prepared by gentle lysis of spheroplasts in the presence of 0.005 M $MgCl_2$. The incubations were carried out singly and in combination with almost everything known to be required for DNase activity. Activity was checked over a pH range between 4 and 9. In no case could any E_2 induced in vitro DNA degradation be detected, even with molar excesses of E_2. Using equivalent levels of pancreatic DNase, we could show extensive degradation, even under conditions far from optimal. The results, of course, do not preclude the possibility of E_2 requiring a special form of DNA for hydrolysis. However, it did not seem profitable to pursue this type of investigation. Therefore, after a lengthy interlude, we returned to our original hypothesis and attempted to reconstitute E_2 induced DNA degradation in lysozyme spheroplasts. Figure 6 shows the results of reconstitution trials

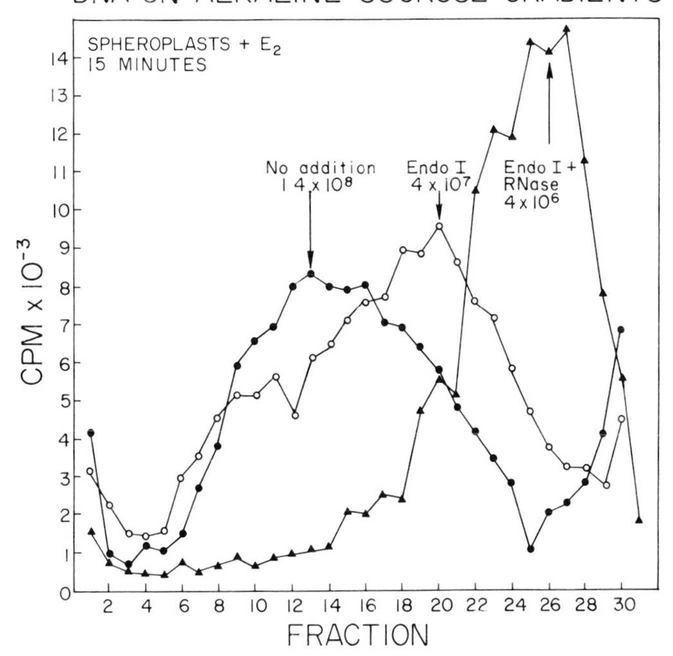

Figure 6 - DNA degradation in spheroplasts treated with colicin E_2 and endonuclease I. Alkaline sucrose gradients for 90 minutes at 35,000 rpm. Colicin E_2 only (●—●). Colicin E_2 + Endo I (o—o). Colicin E_2 + endo I + pancreatic RNase (▲—▲).

done with saturating amounts of E_2. DNA degradation in the spheroplast preparations was analyzed by performing alkaline sucrose gradient centrifugation on aliquots of the DNA obtained from spheroplast lysates. The spheroplast DNA was labeled with ^{32}P. The radioactivity measured in the DNA fractions obtained in the alkaline sucrose gradients represents the acid insoluble, alkali resistant ^{32}P fraction of the DNA. Colicin E_2 alone did not induce DNA degradation in the spheroplast preparations. The unincubated or incubated controls and the experimental tubes containing E_2 showed the same DNA peak on alkaline gradients. When a crude preparation of endonuclease I was added to the incubation mixture containing E_2, the single strand molecular weight of the spheroplast DNA shifted from 1.4×10^8 to 4×10^7 daltons after a 15 minute incubation. If pancreatic RNase was also present in the reaction mixture, the peak shifted even more, giving a DNA molecular weight in the range of 4×10^6 daltons. This latter figure is almost the limit size of DNA seen under *in vivo* conditions in normal assay

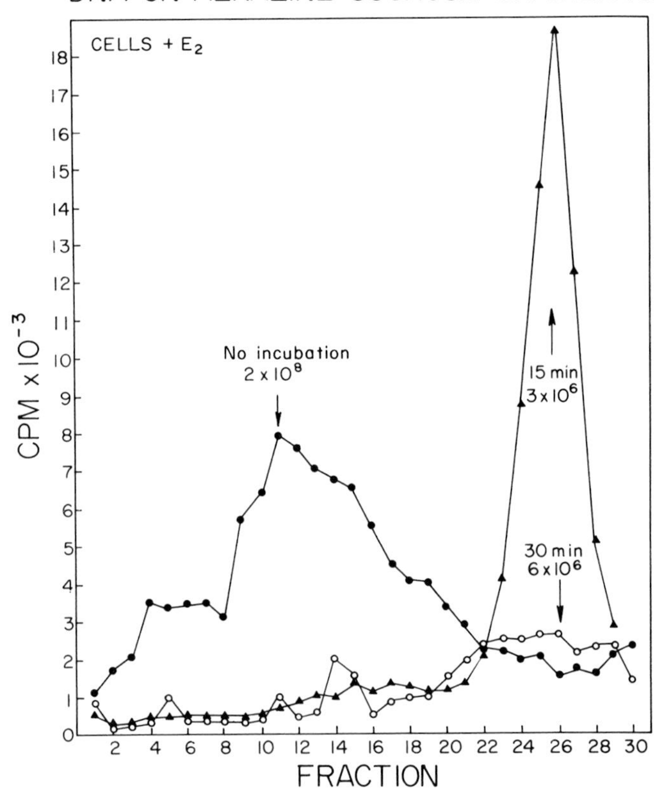

Figure 7 - DNA degradation in normal cells treated with colicin E_2. Alkaline sucrose gradients as Figure 6. No incubation (●—●). Fifteen minutes at 37° (▲—▲). Thirty minutes at 37° (o—o).

cells treated with E_2. Upon further incubation, the DNA in the assay mixtures containing E_2, endonuclease I, and RNase showed little change in molecular weight. However, in the latter case, the DNA peak in alkaline sucrose gradients did become sharper with time. In no case, could any sizable exonuclease activity be detected.

For comparison purposes, Figure 7 shows the extent of DNA degradation in normal cells treated with similar colicin levels. After 15 minutes incubation, these cells have had their DNA degraded to the limit size, and in 30 minutes, most of the DNA has become acid soluble. The DNA that remains, however, is still at the limit size that was reached in 15 minutes.

The endonuclease I which was used for these initial reconstitution studies was obtained as a major contaminant from our crude colicin preparations. For the reconstitution experiments, it had been partially purified by ammonium sulfate fractionation and DEAE Sephadex chromatography. However, the partially purified endonuclease I still contained considerable amounts of colicin E_2. When the levels of endonuclease I in the reconstitution assay were lowered to decrease the E_2 contamination to less than 1 killing unit per spheroplast, it could be shown that there was a requirement for both endonuclease I and for colicin E_2 to induce DNA degradation in spheroplasts. However, under these conditions of low endonuclease activity, it took much longer to obtain the effect (30 minutes as opposed to 15 minutes), and the extent of degradation was less. The levels of endonuclease I added in this instance were only about 5 per cent of the total endonuclease released by the cells during spheroplast formation. Furthermore, the effective concentration of endonuclease was very much less than that which occurs in the periplasmic space since the *in vitro* experiments required measurable volumes in the assay mixtures. Therefore it wasn't surprising that the lag time for DNA degradation was extended and that only limited degradation was observed under these conditions.

Next, a crude extract of endonuclease I was prepared from cells which did not produce colicin E_2 so that the above studies could be repeated with higher levels of endonuclease I free of contamination with E_2. Such experiments would determine if both endonuclease I and colicin E_2 were absolutely necessary for reconstitution. Unfortunately, this symposium session was fast approaching so there was not time to carry out an extensive purification of the new endonuclease I preparation. The enzyme was purified only through an initial ammonium sulfate precipitation step. As a result, there was a very high level of 260nm absorbing material present in the preparation and the endonuclease I activity was strongly inhibited, presumably by RNA. However, using this preparation it was still found that DNA degradation only occurred in spheroplasts when both E_2 and endonuclease I were present (Figure 8). Spheroplasts which were incubated only with colicin E_2 or only endonuclease I showed no DNA degradation. The DNA peak on alkaline gradients gave an average molecular weight of 1.2×10^8 daltons when the spheroplasts were incubated singly with either E_2 or endonuclease I. However, the combination of E_2 and endonuclease I together produced a DNA species having an average molecular weight of $4. \times 10^7$ daltons. When pancreatic RNase was also present, somewhat more degradation occurred although the limit size of the DNA core was not yet reached. In fact, the presence of pancreatic RNase seemed to remove the requirement for colicin E_2 because RNase plus endonuclease I induced as much DNA degradation as did mixtures of colicin E_2 and endonuclease I plus or minus RNase.

Neutral gradients were attempted for each of these samples but quantitative release of the DNA from the rapidly precipitating membrane complex could not be obtained. As a result, it is not yet known whether we are observing single or double strand cleavages in these recombination experiments. We also have not been able to measure reliable exonucle-

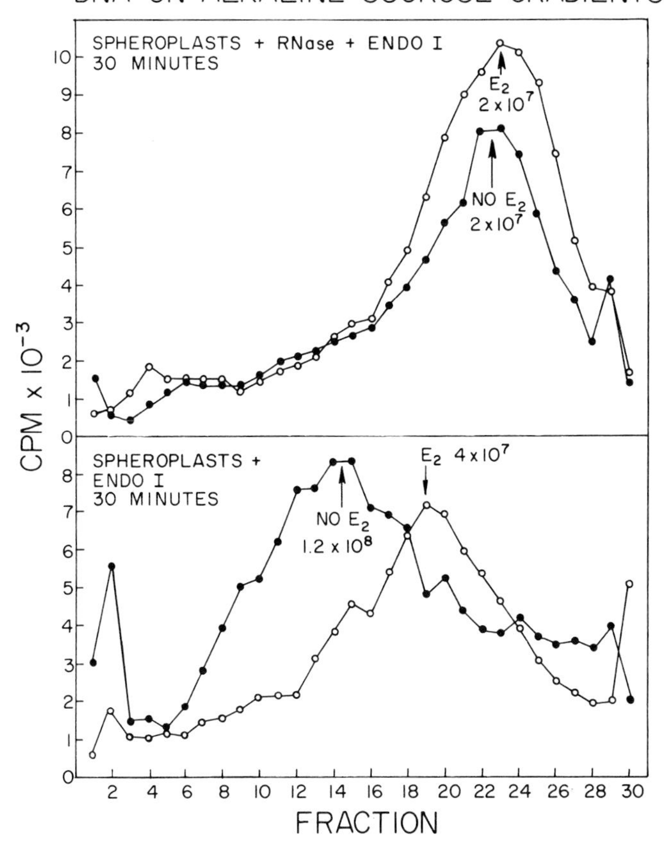

Figure 8 - DNA degradation in spheroplasts treated with E_2 and endonuclease I. Alkaline sucrose gradients as figure 6. Bottom graph: endonuclease I (●—●), endonuclease I + E_2 (o—o). Top graph: endonuclease I + pancreatic RNase (●—●), endonuclease I + pancreatic RNase + colicin E_2 (o—o).

ase activity in any of the samples, but we have not had time to optimize the conditions used.

The important thing to note from these reconstitution experiments is that crude endonuclease I plus E_2 produces DNA degradation in spheroplasts while neither one will do it separately. The E_2-endonuclease I induced degradation produces internal cleavages, and the activity appears to stop near the same limit molecular weight as seen in whole cells treated with E_2 alone. The possibility exists of course that another endonuclease may also be present in these fairly crude preparations. We do know that a ribonuclease is present in the crude endonuclease preparation and in fact we can even observe, in the presence of E_2, an extensive degradation of high molecular weight spheroplast RNA. Again RNA degradation in the spheroplasts requires both E_2 and a component in the crude endonuclease preparation. We have not yet had time to identify either the RNA involved or the RNase, although we feel it is probably RNase I which is responsible.

These experiments do not exclude the possibility that E_2 is a DNase and that E_2 is being complemented by something other than endonuclease I in the crude endonuclease fractions which are used for reconstitution. Such a hypothesis would require that the activated E_2 show the same mechanism of degradation as the uninhibited endonuclease I. Further purification of the endonuclease preparation is planned in order to perform more definitive experiments. A pure endonuclease preparation should allow us to decide between all of these possibilities.

We also attempted to see if E_2 is required for or would stimulate DNA degradation by endonuclease I in cell lysates. Figure 9 shows that high E_2 levels do enhance DNA degradation slightly as can be seen by comparing the curves with high and low levels of E_2. Again, in this case, pancreatic RNase did a much better job of activating endonuclease I than did E_2. However, the results of this experiment are difficult to assess because extensive DNA degradation is also being carried out by other enzymes present in the crude lysates. All of the incubated controls gave DNA peaks approximately like the peak labeled E_2 and RNase in Figure 9. The unincubated lysates showed DNA having a molecular weight of 1.4×10^8 daltons.

When we first compared the results showing the activation of endonuclease I by colicin E_2 and by

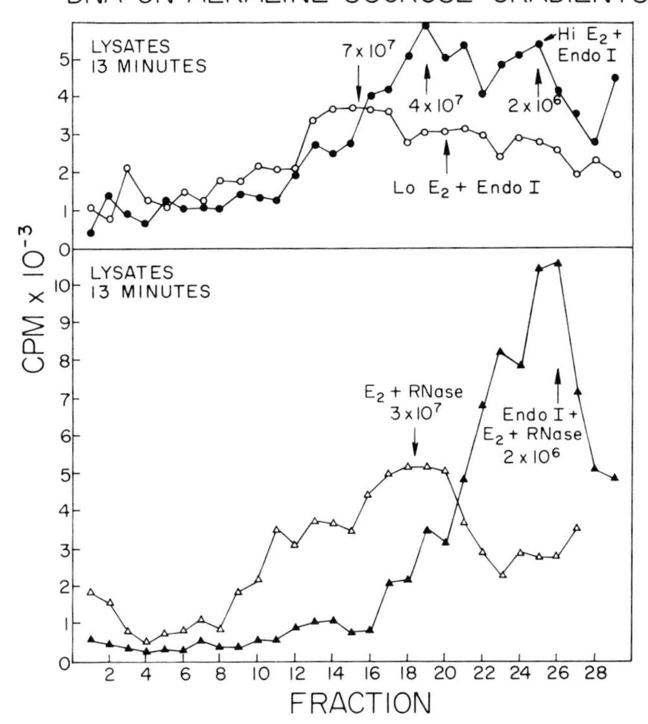

Figure 9 - DNA degradation in cell lysates treated with endonuclease I and E_2. Alkaline sucrose gradients as figure 6. Endonuclease I + low E_2 (o—o), Endonuclease I + high E_2 (●—●), Endonuclease I + high E_2 + pancreatic RNase (▲—▲), high E_2 + RNase (△—△).

pancreatic RNase in the spheroplast system, it seemed as if the E_2 might be acting as an RNase and removing inhibitory RNA from endonuclease I. However, we have not been able to demonstrate this type of activation *in vitro* using crude endonuclease I plus E_2, either with poly dAT or pure *E. coli* DNA as substrate. Two different assay procedures were used in the attempts to detect *in vitro* activation. Both the formation of acid soluble material from ^{32}P labeled DNA and the monitoring of the molecular weight of DNA on alkaline sucrose gradients failed to detect in vitro activation. An interesting observation which came from this cell free system was that the endonuclease I activated by the RNase appears to have lost the ability to stop at the 2 x 10^6 molecular weight limit size for DNA as seen with spheroplasts. The DNA in the cell free system is degraded to pieces smaller than 1 x 10^6 daltons and, of course, to acid soluble material. These observations indicate that the activity occurring in the spheroplasts and cells is highly modified in comparison to that seen in cell free systems.

From all of this evidence, we must conclude that endonuclease I is involved in the E_2 induced degradation of cellular DNA. Initially, we postulated that E_2 might reverse a transport system which could be used by the cell to remove the endonuclease I from its place of manufacture in the cytoplasm (2). However, we must now also consider the possibility that E_2 causes the release of the inhibitory RNA from the endonuclease I and that the active endonuclease is then transported into the cell or inserted on the membrane such that it can degrade cytoplasmic DNA. This latter hypothesis is attractive in light of the fact that colicins E_2 and E_3 are very similar molecules and theoretically should act by similar mechanisms. In this latter hypothesis both E_2 and E_3 could be RNases endowed with high specificity. However, whether E_2 and E_3 are themselves ribonucleases, or whether they activate cellular enzymes is a moot question at this time.

References

1. M. Nomura, Ann. Rev. Microbiol. 21, 257 (1967).
2. R. Almendinger and L. P. Hager, Nature New Biology 235, 199 (1972).
3. A. Maeda and M. Nomura, J. Bact. 91, 685 (1966).
4. M. Nomura, Cold Spring Harbor Symp. Quant. Biol. 28, 315 (1963).
5. B. L. Reynolds and P. R. Reeves, Biochem. Biophys. Res. Comm. 11, 140 (1963).

6. M. Nomura and A. Maeda, Zentr. Bakteriol. Parasitenk. Abt. I. Orig. 196, 216 (1965).
7. M. Nomura, Proc. Natl. Acad. Sci. 52, 1514 (1964).
8. E. M. Holland and I. B. Holland, J. Gen. Microbiol. 64, 223 (1970).
9. M. Obinata and D. Mizuno, Biochim. Biophys. Acta 199, 330 (1970).
10. P. Ringrose, Biochim. Biophys. Acta 213, 320 (1970).
11. L. S. Saxe and S. E. Luria, Bact. Proc., 50 (1971).
12. B. L. Reynolds and P. R. Reeves, J. Bact. 100, 301 (1969).
13. T. Beppu and K. Arima, J. Biochem. 70, 263 (1971).
14. K. Nose and D. Mizuno, J. Biochem. 64, 1 (1968).
15. K. Nose, D. Mizuno and H. Ozeki, Biochim. Biophys. Acta 119, 636 (1966).
16. A. Yamai, T. Beppu and K. Arima, Agr. Biol. Chem. 34, 149 (1970).
17. J. Konisky and M. Nomura, J. Mol. Biol. 26, 181 (1967).
18. H. C. Neu and L. A. Heppel, Biochem. Biophys. Res. Comm. 17, 215 (1964).
19. H. C. Neu and L. A. Heppel, J. Biol. Chem. 240, 3685 (1965).
20. C. Cordonnier and G. Bernardi, Biochem. Biophys. Res. Comm. 20, 555 (1965).
21. N. G. Nossal and L. A. Heppel, J. Biol. Chem. 241, 3055 (1966).
22. J. Done, C. D. Shorey, J. P. Lake and J. K. Pollak, Biochem. J. 96, 27C (1965).
23. V. M. Kushnarev and T. A. Smirnova, Can. J. Microbiol. 12, 605 (1966).
24. I. Nisonson, M. Tannenbaum and H. C. Neu, J. Bact. 100, 1083 (1969).
25. B. K. Wetzel, S. S. Spicer, H. F. Dvorak and L. A. Heppel, J. Bact. 104, 529 (1970).
26. I. R. Beacham, E. Yagil, K. Beacham and R. H. Pritchard, FEBS Letters 16, 77 (1971).

27. I. R. Lehman, G. G. Roussos and E. A. Pratt, J. Biol. Chem. 237, 819 (1962).
28. I. R. Lehman, G. G. Roussos and E. A. Pratt, J. Biol. Chem. 237, 829 (1962).
29. A. DeWaard and I. R. Lehman, ed. G. L. Cantoni and D. R. Davies, Procedures in Nucleic Acid Research, 122, Harper and Row, N.Y. (1966).
30. C. Paoletti, J. B. LePecq, and I. R. Lehman, J. Mol. Biol. 55, 75 (1971).
31. E. Melgar and D. A. Goldthwait, J. Biol. Chem. 243, 4401 (1968).
32. F. W. Studier, J. Mol. Biol. 11, 373 (1965).
33. W. Goebel and D. R. Helinski, Biochemistry 9, 4793 (1970).
34. T. Beppu and K. Arima, J. Bact. 93, 80 (1967).
35. E. H. Cota-Robles, J. Bact. 85, 499 (1963).
36. H. F. Dvorak, B. K. Wetzel and L. A. Heppel, J. Bact. 104, 543 (1970).
37. L. A. Heppel, Science 156, 1451 (1967).
38. Y. Anraku and L. A. Heppel, J. Biol. Chem. 242, 2561 (1967).
39. L. Leive, Biochem. Biophys. Res. Comm. 21, 290 (1965).
40. H. C. Neu, D. F. Ashman and T. D. Price, Biochem. Biophys. Res. Comm. 25, 615 (1966).
41. H. C. Neu, D. F. Ashman and T. D. Price, J. Bact. 93, 1360 (1967).
42. L. Leive, and V. Kollin, Biochem. Biophys. Res. Comm. 28, 229 (1967).
43. L. Leive, V. K. Shovlin and S. E. Mergenhagen, J. Biol. Chem. 243, 6384 (1968).
44. H. Dürwald and H. Hoffman-Berling, J. Mol. Biol. 34, 331 (1968).
45. R. Levisohn, J. Konisky and M. Nomura, J. Bact. 96, 811 (1967).
46. T. Boon, Proc. Natl. Acad. Sci. 68, 2421 (1971).
47. T. Boon, Proc. Natl. Acad. Sci. 69, 549 (1972).
48. C. M. Bowman, J. Sidikaro and M. Nomura, Nature New Biology 234, 133 (1971).
49. C. M. Bowman, FEBS Letters 22, 73 (1972).
50. T. Beppu and K. Arima, Biochim. Biophys. Acta

219, 512 (1970).
51. T. Beppu and K. Arima, Biochim. Biophys. Acta 262, 453 (1972).

SUBJECT INDEX